Languages and Genes in Northwestern China and Adjacent Regions

Dan Xu · Hui Li
Editors

Languages and Genes in Northwestern China and Adjacent Regions

Springer

Editors
Dan Xu
Département Chine
INALCO
Paris Cedex
France

Hui Li
School of Life Sciences
Fudan University
Shanghai
China

ISBN 978-981-10-4168-6 ISBN 978-981-10-4169-3 (eBook)
DOI 10.1007/978-981-10-4169-3

Library of Congress Control Number: 2017934633

Printed on acid-free paper

This Springer imprint is published by Springer Nature
The registered company is Springer Nature Singapore Pte Ltd.
The registered company address is: 152 Beach Road, #21-01/04 Gateway East, Singapore 189721, Singapore

Preface

This book is the result of a four-year-long collaboration between linguists and geneticists working on the project ANR-12-BSH2-0004-01 *Do languages and genes correlate?—A case study in Northwestern China* funded by a grant from a French research fund, the *Agence Nationale de la Recherche* (ANR). Numerous researchers from different institutions around the world have taken part in this project and have contributed to two collective works. In addition to work performed at the *Centre de Recherches Linguistiques sur l'Asie Orientale* (CRLAO-CNRS) and the *Institut National des Langues et Civilisations Orientales* (INALCO) in France, genetic data in the target zone were collected and analyzed by Fudan University, Lanzhou University, and the Gansu Institute of Political Science and Law in China, providing a solid framework for this project. Linguists from the Institute of Ethnology and Anthropology at the Chinese Academy of Social Sciences (CASS), the University of Ethnology, Tsinghua University in China, the Chinese University of Hong Kong, Doshisha University in Kyoto, Japan, and St. Mary's College of Maryland, USA, have completed different work related to language contact in China. Twenty-one articles have been included in a book entitled *Yuyan jiechu yu yuyan bianyi* [language contact and variation] (which will be published by Shangwu yinshuguan [Commercial Press] in China). As the title indicates, language contact constitutes the main topic of the project's first book. The present volume *Languages and Genes in Northwestern China and Adjacent Regions* mainly focuses on (non-)correlation between languages and genes in Northwest China. Ten authors have offered their works to this book. Warm thanks go to these institutions and specially to these researchers. Without their work, the results of our interdisciplinary approach would never have been available to those who might make use of them.

Today, it is becoming common for molecular anthropologists, archeologists, and linguists to work together to explore the social sciences. If we are not aware of the historical period we live in, we will miss the opportunity of learning from other researchers, depriving ourselves of the pleasure of knowing research domains other than our own.

Our final thanks go to Craig Baker who has proofread our manuscript with patience.

Paris, France
Shanghai, China
December 2016

Dan Xu
Hui Li

Contents

Introduction

Dan Xu and Hui Li

The present book entitled ***Languages and Genes in Northwestern China and Adjacent Regions*** consists of an investigation of language contact, focused on Northwestern China. What is new in the book is that the research is not limited to a linguistic perspective but is extended to an interdisciplinary approach, exploiting research results from different domains.

Human history is very complicated and can only be fully examined by cross-disciplinary studies. Study from just one field can only demonstrate one side of the story. Linguistic studies can find cultural contact among populations, but cannot determine whether people migrated and intermixed, which can be proven by genetic studies, and completed by archeological, anthropological and historical research. In other words, linguistic data is sometimes hard to interpret without further information from other areas. Breakthroughs in linguistic research require a new approach. Few linguists have consciously taken advantage of recent results from other sciences such as biology. The present work attempts to break the barrier between human sciences and natural sciences to reconsider the diversity of languages on the basis of current research results from linguistics, genetics and other domains. The work focuses on Northern and Northwestern China, without neglecting the northern area beyond China's borders. It is of great interest to find

D. Xu (✉)
Institut National des Langues et Civilisations Orientales (INALCO),
63 Rue des Grands Moulins, 75013 Paris, France
e-mail: xusongdan@gmail.com

D. Xu
CRLAO (CNRS), Paris, France

H. Li (✉)
MOE Key Laboratory of Contemporary Anthropology, School of Life Sciences,
Fudan University, Shanghai 200438, People's Republic of China
e-mail: 39232074@qq.com

D. Xu and H. Li (eds.), *Languages and Genes in Northwestern China and Adjacent Regions*, DOI 10.1007/978-981-10-4169-3_1

out when and how the divergence of languages and genes began and when and how language and gene admixture and replacement occurred.

Modern humans migrated out of Africa around 70 thousand years ago, and spread rapidly over the rest of the world (Underhill et al. 2000). Adapting to diverse environments in different regions, humans evolved into eight regional groups. East Asia is one large group among them. East Asia is a sub-region of Asia, with a vast and diverse landscape (Sagart et al. 2005). Concerning the extension of cultures and genetics, we usually include the flanking region of Siberia and Southeast Asia within East Asia. About one third of the world's population lives in East Asia, and more than 1500 languages from ten families (Altaic[1], Austroasiatic, Austronesian, Tai-Kadai, Hmong-Mien, Sino-Tibetan, Uralic, Yeniseian, Palaesiberian, and Indo-European) are spoken in East Asia (Li and Jin 2015), which make this region one of the world's most important places for studying human evolution, genetic diversity, and interrelationships between genetics and cultures of human populations.

The correlation between genetic structure and linguistic classification is not inevitable, but is observed consistently among East Asian populations. A good sample of research was published in *Science* in 2009, showing that overall genomic diversity was clearly associated with linguistic families (HUGO Pan-Asian SNP Consortium 2009). Almost all populations whose languages were of the same linguistic family clustered together in the same genetic clade. This study collected wide samples from East Asia, including populations speaking Austronesian, Austroasiatic, Tai-Kadai, Hmong-Mien, Sino-Tibetan, Indo-European, and Altaic. Besides the genetic clustering of the linguistic families, the relationships among families were also informative. A phylogenetic tree was constructed with a chimpanzee genome as the root. The African, South Asian, and East Asian branches diverged in sequence, supporting the African origin of modern humans. Within the East Asian branch, the Austronesian clade was closest to the root, and then the Austroasiatic, Tai-Kadai, Hmong-Mien, Sino-Tibetan, and Korean-Japanese branches. This means that the early peopling of East Asia was from the south. However, this phylogenetic structure did not match the history of the linguistic families. For example, the Austronesian people relocated from southeastern China to island Southeast Asia around 6000 years ago (Li et al. 2007, 2008), which means this group was not originally in southernmost East Asia. Therefore, the current genetic situation must have come from cultural assimilation of the indigenous populations in Southeast Asia. One solid piece of evidence is that the Negrito populations of the Philippines and Malaysia were situated inside the Austronesian clade, even though they could not have spoken an Austronesian language for long. In conclusion, we suggest that, at a larger genomic scale, genetic consistency within a linguistic family probably comes from frequent gene flow within the family, and the genetic diversification between families from cultural barriers between families.

---

[1]The term "Altaic" has always been debated in the linguistic community.

While most of the linguistic families showed genetic consistency, the Altaic family showed a pronounced genetic inconsistency (Karafet et al. 2002). The Turkic subfamily is quite far from the other subfamilies in both genetics and linguistics (Kharkov et al. 2007; Zhou and Xie 2008; Shou and Xiao 2010). In the whole genomic phylogenetic tree, Turkic populations are distributed between Indo-European and East Asian groups. Therefore, we conclude that Turkic was an admixture group between Eastern and Western Eurasians.

Whole genomic analyses can only exhibit the integrative structure of Paleolithic dispersal and Neolithic assimilation within families but not the relationships among the groups speaking certain linguistic families. Fortunately, much research has demonstrated that the Y chromosome carries information about interfamily relationships (Stumpf and Goldstein 2001). In a worldwide illustration, Forster and Renfrew (2011) pointed out that Y-chromosome DNA types are related to language in Sub-Saharan Africa, Iceland, India, Papua New Guinea, and the Southwest of North America. Such correlations are not observed for mtDNA, which is inherited from the mother. In East Asia, this kind of correlation between Y chromosome and language is even stronger. Almost all of the linguistic families have been investigated for Y chromosomes. Interestingly, genetic resemblance was observed between three pairs of linguistic families: Austronesian and Tai-Kadai speakers have a high frequency of Y haplogroup O1 (Li et al. 2008), Hmong-Mien and Austroasiatic speakers comprise a unique haplogroup O3-M7 (Cai et al. 2011), and Yeniseian and Palaesiberian speakers have a high frequency of haplogroup Q (Karafet et al. 2002; Kharkov et al. 2007). We then presume that people from each pair of linguistic families might share a recent ancestral population.

As is assumed in linguistics, the large linguistic family might have originated no earlier than 8000–10,000 years ago at the beginning of the Neolithic Age. The Neolithic Age societies in East Asia were led by males who were also carrying languages. For a linguistic family to expand to a large population scale, there must be a large area and a long time for this family to be spoken. Therefore, there might be certain Neolithic cultural contexts related to the origin of linguistic family. Fortunately, this hypothesis is supported by Y chromosome studies (Li et al. 2007). For example, ethnological studies suggest an origin in Southeastern China for Tai-Kadai and Austronesian families. In the Neolithic Age, the Liangzhu cultural context was distributed in this region. The human remains from Liangzhu sites belong to Y haplogroup O1, which is the unique haplogroup of Tai-Kadai and Austronesian speakers. Similar linkages were found between the Daxi culture context and Hmong-Mien/Austroasiatic speakers in the central Yangtze region with high frequency of haplogroup O3-M7, and Longshan culture and Sino-Tibetan speakers in the Yellow River region with high frequency of haplogroup O3-M134. These Neolithic cultural contexts might have served as substrates for the co-evolution of genetic confederates and linguistic families. Thus, to further understand the evolutionary history of linguistic families, interdisciplinary studies among linguistics, genetics, and archaeology are most important.

Linguistics became one of the most rigorous branches of human sciences with Saussure's (1857–1913) work. Inspired by the natural sciences, linguistics segments a speech chain into optimally analyzable units: phoneme, morpheme, phrase, paradigm, synchrony, diachrony, etc. In other words, linguistics converts a continuum into discrete elements in order to objectively observe them. In today's information age, there is a tendency to combine different research disciplines, since the development of computer science and technology allows us to associate different domains. Research requires a microscopic approach as well as a macroscopic one. Human sciences research is only promising when using results from other disciplines; it can have breakthroughs only with the associated efforts of different realms. In this sense, much work needs to be done in human sciences and many gaps need to be filled.

In his famous book *On the Origin of Species* published in 1859, Charles Darwin already believed that "If we possessed a perfect pedigree of mankind, a genealogical arrangement of the races of man would afford the best classification of the various languages now spoken throughout the world; and if all extinct languages, and all intermediate and slowly changing dialects had to be included, such an arrangement would, I think, be the only possible one" (Chap. 13). As the same period of Darwin, a linguist August Schleicher established a first linguistic tree to compare distances between languages. Actually, languages and genes display several similarities in their evolution (see Pagel 2009). With great progress of molecular biology since the 1980s, more and more research has combined these two domains.

Historians, anthropologists, archaeologists and linguists have long been interested in Northwestern China, including the Silk Road located in China (in Gansu, Qinghai and Xinjiang). For the past several decades, linguists and other human science researchers have combined their efforts to better understand the social, anthropological, and linguistic phenomena in this region. It is an anthropological corridor where numerous historical migrations have taken place. Nomadic pastoralist life patterns confronted farming expansions, and Eastern and Western ethnic peoples exchanged their merchandise, languages and cultures, and even their genes. In this area, Nestorianism, Buddhism and Islam opposed each other, engaging people in uninterruptible wars. Conquerors as well as victims passed through this corridor speaking their own languages as well as others' languages. The linguistic situation was and still is complex due to these historic factors. Three language families coexisted and had contact even before the existence of the Silk Road: the Sino-Tibetan, Altaic and Indo-European families (the latter consisting of the Tocharian language, which went extinct around the 9th century, as well as Tajik and Russian spoken today in the extreme west of Xinjiang).

Northwestern China is an area inhabited by different ethnic groups: Chinese (Han), Hui (Muslims), Santa (Dongxiang), Bao'an (Baonan), Monguor (Tu), Eastern Yugur, Western Yugur, Uyghur, Salar, Amdo Tibetan, Kazakh, Kirgiz, Uzbek, Tatar, Sibo, etc. From a linguistic point of view, the Santa, Bao'an, Monguor and Eastern Yugur languages belong to the Mongolic group of the Altaic family (still disputed), while the rest, except the Amdo Tibetan groups which are classified within the Tibeto-Burman group in the Sino-Tibetan family, are part of the Turkic group in the same family. These people speak different languages, and the Chinese language spoken next to or surrounded by them has undergone dramatic changes. The present book will focus on language evolution between the border of Gansu and Qinghai. Manchu, a dying language belonging to the Tungusic group, will be also studied to complete our understanding of language replacement.

1 Organization of the Book

The paper "*Correlation between genetic structure and linguistic phylogeny in East Asia*" by Yunzhi Huang and Hui Li provides a general landscape of correlation between population and languages in East Asia. Both languages and genes can serve as an important clue to the history of human populations (Cavalli-Sforza 1997, 2000). Most linguists believe that languages within a certain linguistic family have a common origin within the past 10 thousand years, which also fits perfectly with Neolithic archaeological evidence for the advent of agriculture in each region (Cavalli-Sforza et al. 1994). Thus, Bellwood (2013) proposed a farming/language dispersal hypothesis that male farmers replaced the neighboring hunter-gatherers, leading to a male-bias language replacement. This hypothesis has been proven by genetic evidence. Linguistic families show a strong association with Y-chromosomal diversity but not with mtDNA variations (Forster and Renfrew 2011). In East Asia, we did find that linguistic families are well associated with Y chromosome diversity. Most families have their dominant Y lineages, for instance the Y chromosome haplogroup O3-M134 in Sino-Tibetan speakers, O2-M95 and O3-M7 in Hmong-Mien and Austro-Asiatic speakers, O1-M119 in Tai-Kadai and Austronesian speakers, N-TAT in Uralic speakers, Q-M242 in Yeniseian speakers, and C3-M217 in Altaic(Tungusic-Mongolian) speakers (Li and Jin 2015). Thus, Y-chromosomal lineages of a population can sometimes predict their linguistic affiliation. Furthermore, according to the similarity in the Y chromosome profiles, there are four pairs of congenetic families, that is, Austronesian and Tai-Kadai, Mon-Khmer and Hmong-Mien, Sino-Tibetan and Uralic, Yeniseian and Palaesiberian, demonstrating the substantial early language contact and gene flow between these ancient populations. Notably, between approximately 4000 and 2000 kya, Tai-Kadai, Hmong-Mien, Sino-Tibetan, and Yeniseian languages transformed into tonal analytic languages, becoming quite different from the other four (Wang 2000). There must be some social or biological factors which induced the transformations at that time, a topic worthy of more linguistic and genetic research.

The paper "*Genetic perspective on language replacement in Siberia*" by Lanhai Wei and Hui Li treats language replacement in the light of biological research. Recent instances of language replacement may have left pronounced genetic effects, and thus warrant molecular anthropological investigation. However, little work has been done towards this goal. Previous research showed that diversity in Y-chromosome haplogroups (indicating male lineages) of Siberian populations is low, and populations using languages of the same group tend to share the same predominant paternal lineages (Karafet et al. 2002; Kharkov et al. 2007; Shou and Xiao 2010). To study the origin and diffusion of linguistic groups and recent instances of language replacement in Siberia, Lanhai Wei and Hui Li conducted a comprehensive comparison of Y-chromosome haplogroup frequencies among 131 populations in Siberia and neighboring regions. The authors summarized that N1c-M46 and N2a1-P43 are two founding paternal lineages in Uralic-speaking populations. For the Ket population, the only surviving Yeniseian-speaking group, the predominant lineage is Q-L330. The founding paternal lineages in Mongolic-speaking populations were identified as C3*-Star Cluster and C3d-M407, while the only predominant lineage in Tungusic-speaking populations is C3c-M48. For Turkic-speaking populations, no predominant lineage was observed. This article proposes that language replacement has occurred when the major paternal lineage of a population is not the predominant one within their linguistic group, but is instead a downstream sub-clade of a lineage which recently expanded from another linguistic group. The authors argue that after the immigration and admixture of ancient populations, language replacement may have occurred in the Selkups, Tuvan, Kyrgyz, Kazak, Khakassian, Shors, Yakuts, various Mongolic-speaking populations, and in the Aisin Gioro clan of the Manchu ethnicity. This research indicates that accurate genetic dating can help to explore the unknown admixture history of populations, as well as the origin and diffusion/replacement of their languages. This powerful new approach can be applied to other linguistic groups in other parts of the world.

The work "*The Silk Road: language and population admixture and replacement*" by Dan Xu and Shaoqing Wen focusses on languages and populations on the Silk Road within China. This paper investigates the (non-)correlation between languages and genes on the Silk Road. It is expected to provide a clear picture of human migration history between Central Asia and East Asia. Diachronic linguistics needs new ways to go beyond its chronological limits. Combining natural sciences and human sciences enables us to overcome the limits of traditional methodology in historical linguistics. In light of biological and archeological research results, where dating is based on concrete materials, the investigation will trace language ancestry on the Silk Road over the same timescales. Comparing language distance based on ethnic genetic distance will help us to reconstruct different historical periods during which dispersing populations, bearers of diverse genes, also spread their languages. Why are language-gene correlations often broken on the Silk Road? As has been mentioned, the Silk Road is occupied by different ethnic groups. The paper will take eight representative languages (East Yugur, Tu, Dongxiang and Bao'an from the Mongolic language group, and Uyghur, Kazakh, West Yugur and Salar from the Turkic group) in studying language admixture and replacement with a biological background. It will show that some languages are the result of admixture over several centuries, and some others are newborn languages, like their populations: they completely replaced other languages due to important historical migrations of their ancestors. Two models of language replacement will be studied. (1) the Elite Dominance model, initially proposed by Renfrew (1987); (2) the Cultural Dominance model, put forth by this article, which will complete the first model.

"*Relationship between Altaic speaking populations and their languages viewed from Y chromosomes*" by Shaoqing Wen, Xiaodong Xie and Dan Xu studies languages and populations at the border of Gansu and Qinghai. Gansu province is located in Northwest China, between the Mongolian plateau, the Loess plateau and the Tibetan plateau. It is a region of linguistic, cultural and genetic mixing of various ethnic groups speaking various Sinitic and non-Sinitic languages. Within the historical context of East-West exchange, present-day populations in this area show a high level of both linguistic and genetic diversity, indicating that their languages and genetic makeup may be associated with complex processes of linguistic contact and population admixture (Zhou and Xie 2008). The region is rich in human genetic and linguistic resources. Most of the ethnic groups inhabiting in this region belong to the Altaic linguistic family. Nevertheless, little is known about the relationship between the genetic makeup of Altaic speaking populations and their languages. We collected 964 male samples from 20 ethnic groups in Northwestern China, and surveyed 12 Y-chromosomal biallelic markers to reconstruct the paternal architecture. The result of multidimensional scaling analysis indicates that the Tungusic group and Turkic group show large genetic distances to each other, and the Mongolian group was close to the Tungusic group, somewhat apart from the Turkic group. Principal component analyses also confirm this result. A phylogenetic tree signified a general association between Y chromosomes of Altaic speaking populations and their linguistic affiliations, revealing a coevolution of Y chromosome diversity and languages in Northwest China.

The paper "*Formation of a "Mixed Language" in Northwest China-The Case of Tangwang*" by Dan Xu and Shaoqing Wen studies the Tangwang language from an interdisciplinary perspective. Within the historical context of East-West exchanges, present-day populations in this area show a high level of both linguistic and genetic diversity, indicating that their languages and genetic makeup may be associated with complex processes of linguistic contact and population admixture. The authors try to combine a linguistic approach with a biological one, to better understand the coevolution of language and genes. The Tangwang people and their language are an ideal model for studying language contact and formation of a new population. In this study, 151 male samples were first collected from 5 family clans (with surnames Tang, Wang, Zhang, Yang and Zao) in the town of Tangwang in Linxia Hui Autonomous Prefecture, Gansu province, to trace the origin and demographic history of the Tangwang people, and then 96 linguistic features of the Tangwang language and other reference languages in China were investigated. The results show that: (1) Almost all the clans have dominant paternal lineages associated with different origins; (2) the times to most recent common ancestor of the 5 clans coincide with the records of local settlement history; (3) based on 96 linguistic features, the Tangwang language tends to cluster with Sinitic languages rather than with non-Sinitic languages. Overall, the authors employ the principle of language, Y chromosome and clan co-evolution to reconstruct the formation of a mixed population and their languages, and to further study the relationships between language contact and population admixture.

The work "*Present Y chromosomes refute the Roma/Gypsy origin of the Xuejiawan people in Northwest China*" by Shaoqing Wen, Dan Xu, Hongbing Yao and Hui Li examines a language discovered in the 1940s and considered to be a "mysterious language". Since a journalist reported in 1947 that the Xuejiawan people of Northwestern China had an ancient Gypsy origin, these so-called eastern gypsies have attracted wide publicity (Xu 2016). Nonetheless, regarding the ethnic origins of the Xuejiawan people, scholars from different disciplines have stuck to their opinions, which mainly comprise three popular hypotheses (the ancient Gypsy origin hypothesis, the Northern Chinese origin hypothesis, and the southern Hmong-Mien origin hypothesis). To address this issue, an interdisciplinary investigation was carried out by a joint team formed by Chinese geneticists and a French linguist in Xuejiawan village, Yongdeng County, Gansu Province. The results of genetic and genealogical investigations, which involved 118 male individuals from 4 locations, from a set of representative clans (Liu 刘, Liu 柳, Gao 高 and He 何), show that no Western Y chromosomal lineages have been observed in the Xuejiawan people. Moreover, a linguistic comparison of the mysterious Xuejiawan language, spoken by residents of Xuejiawan, with other potentially associated languages found that this language was a kind of argot, called *Shaoju* in Chinese, rather than a non-Han language. The previous literature treats it as a mysterious non-Han language, or even a language of Gypsies who migrated to China. The article shows with abundant proof that many words have been derived from various gang languages. The earliest date to the Song Dynasty. Many *Shaoju* words are innovations based on existing words from different periods. Their phonology, morphology and syntax have to be classified into the Chinese language system even though a few words do come from non-Han languages. Overall, a Gypsy origin cannot be accepted as true due to the paternal gene pool. The wide-ranging linguistic comparison also supports this viewpoint. Taken together, these suggest that the extant Xuejiawan people are more likely to be a subgroup of the Chinese majority Han.

The article "*A comparative analysis of the case system in some Northwestern Sinitic languages*" by Alain Peyraube reexamines the case system recently formed in Northwestern China. The Qinghai-Gansu border region in China (the western part of Qinghai province and the southern part of Gansu province) contains several languages descended from at least four different language taxa: Sinitic, Tibeto-Burman (Amdo Tibetan), Turkic, and Mongolic. Given the frequent contact and intermarriage of Han (Chinese) peoples and Altaic and Tibetan peoples since the beginning of the common era, large scale linguistic contact has inevitably occurred during various periods. It is not surprising that taken individually, most of the region's languages do not seem to conform to their language family's typical typological profile: each has a set of linguistic features which seem to be historically drawn from more than one source. Moreover, if we compare the structural features (especially syntactic features) of the languages throughout the region, we find that they are shared by most of the local language varieties. Thus, there appears to be a regional typological coherence, which can be considered to be a prototypical *Sprachbund*, or *linguistic area*. This paper will examine one of the most characteristic syntactic properties of the languages, namely the case system of the following Sinitic languages: Hezhou [or Linxia], Tangwang, Wutun, and Gangou, which have sometimes been viewed as 'mixed languages.' An answer to the following main questions will be tentatively suggested in the conclusion: Do these languages really have case suffixes (cases are a morphological notion), or do they simply have thematic roles expressed by postpositions (thematic roles are a semantic notion)? Is there really a Qinghai-Gansu linguistic area? Can these Sinitic languages be characterized as 'mixed' languages?

Finally, the work "*The decline of Manchu in its contact with late Qing Chinese—A case study of several editions of Qingwen Zhiyao*" by Meilan Zhang and Jin Qi compares the vocabulary of Manchu through 6 different version of the *Qingwen Zhiyao* (清文指要) to understand the decline of the Manchu language and its replacement by Mandarin (Standard Chinese) over one century. It investigates and compares the vocabulary in the Manchu-Chinese bilingual textbook *Qingwen Zhiyao* with that in 6 different Chinese versions of *Qingwen Zhiyao* written between 1830 and 1920. It is found that the earlier Chinese translations of *Qingwen Zhiyao* were influenced by the Manchu language to a great extent. Some transliterated Manchu words of appellation remained in the earlier Chinese translations, as well as some features of the interlanguage caused by language contact. But most of them disappeared in later Chinese versions, like *Tanlunpian* in *Yu yen tzu erh chi*. It can be concluded that they did not actually enter Chinese. Earlier expressions with Manchu features disappeared as the status of Beijing Mandarin improved. This explains the source of some new uses of Chinese words and the reason for their short duration.

This work comes from a collaboration between two different teams (French and Chinese) composed of linguists and geneticists who worked together for nearly four years. The book takes a novel, interdisciplinary approach, joining linguistic, biological, historical and archeological disciplines. This type of book is currently uncommon, but specialists and lay-readers alike are now aware of the significance of such work. There are numerous books dealing with linguistics or biology separately, but there are few books in which linguists and geneticists work together targeting the same languages and the same populations. This book mainly deals with people and languages in Northwestern China. This region has drawn attention from anthropologists, archaeologists and linguists for several centuries. Over the past several decades, linguists and other human science researchers have combined their efforts to better understand the social, anthropological, and linguistic phenomena in this region, but few investigations seem to take advantage of the recent results from natural sciences such as biology. Many articles in the present work try to combine human science and natural science's approaches to reconsider the diversity of languages in this area based on the results of recent linguistic and genetic research.

References

Amani, Mehdi. 2005. Quelques aspects démographiques relatifs aux langues locales en Iran. In *Contact des Langues dans L'espace arabo-turco-persan*, ed. T. Azadarmaki, C. Balaÿ, and M. Bozdémir, 45–54. Téhéran: Institut français de recherches en Iran.

Atkinson, Quentin D. 2011. Phonemic diversity supports a serial founder effect model of language expansion from Africa. *Science* 332: 346–349.

Bahăr, Mehri, 2005. Interférences linguistiques et culturelles en Iran. In *Contact des Langues dans L'espace arabo-turco-persan*, ed. T. Azadarmaki, C. Balaÿ, and M. Bozdémir, 1–12. Téhéran: Institut français de recherches en Iran.

Bellwood, Peter. 2013. *First migrants*. London: Wiley-Blackwell.

Burlak, S.A. 2013. Languages, DNA, relationship and contacts. *Journal of Language Relationship* Вопросы языкового родства 55–67.

Cai, X., Z. Qin, B. Wen, S. Xu, Y. Wang, Y. Lu, L. Wei, C. Wang, S. Li, X. Huang, L. Jin, and H. Li. 2011. Genographic Consortium: Human migration through bottlenecks from Southeast Asia into East Asia during last glacial maximum revealed by Y chromosomes. *PLoS ONE* 6 (8): e24282.

Cavalli-Sforza, Luigi Luca. 1997. Gene, peoples, and languages. *Proceedings of the National Academy of Sciences of the United States of America* 94: 7719–7724.

Cavalli-Sforza, Luigi Luca. 2000. *Gene, peoples and languages*. London: Penguin Group.

Cavalli-Sforza, Luigi Luca, et al. 1994. *The history and geography of human genes*. Princeton: Princeton University Press.

Darwin, Charles. 1859. *On the origin of species*. London: J. Murray.

Dediu, Dan. 2007. *Non-spurious correlations between genetic and linguistic diversities in the context of human evolution* (Ph.D. dissertation, University of Edinburgh).

Dediu, Dan. 2011. Are languages really independent from genes? If not, what would a genetic bias affecting languages diversity look like? *Human Biology* 83 (2): 279–296.

Dunn, Michael, et al. 2011. Evolved structure of language shows lineage-specific trends in word-order universals. *Nature* (Letter) 1–4.

Forster, P., and C. Renfrew. 2011. Mother tongue and Y chromosomes. *Science* 333: 1390–1391.

HUGO Pan-Asian SNP Consortium. 2009. Mapping human genetic diversity in Asia. *Science* 326: 1541–1545.

Hunley, K.L., et al. 2007. A formal test of linguistic and genetic coevolution in native Central and South America. *American Journal of Physical Anthropology* 132: 622–631.

Karafet, T.M., L.P. Osipova, M.A. Gubina, O.L. Posukh, S.L. Zegura, and M.F. Hammer. 2002. High levels of Y-chromosome differentiation among native Siberian populations and the genetic signature of a boreal hunter-gatherer way of life. *Human Biology* 74: 761–789.

Kharkov, V.N., V.A. Stepanov, O.F. Medvedeva, M.G. Spiridonova, M.I. Voevoda, V.N. Tadinova, and V.P. Puzyrev. 2007. Gene pool differences between northern and southern Altaians inferred from the data on Y-chromosomal haplogroups. *Genetika* 43: 675–687.

Li, Charles N. 1983. Languages in contact in western China. *Papers in East Asian Languages* 1: 31–51.

Li, H., Y. Huang, L.F. Mustavich, F. Zhang, J.Z. Tan, L.E. Wang, J. Qian, M.H. Gao, and L. Jin. 2007. Y chromosomes of prehistoric people along the Yangtze River. *Human Genetics* 122: 383–388.

Li, H., L. Jin. 2015. *Y chromosome and diversification of East Asians*. Shanghai: Shanghai Scientific and Technical Publishers.

Li, H., B. Wen, S.J. Chen, B. Su, P. Pramoonjago, Y. Liu, S. Pan, Z. Qin, W. Liu, X. Cheng, N. Yang, X. Li, D. Tran, D. Lu, M.T. Hsu, R. Deka, S. Marzuki, C.C. Tan, and L. Jin. 2008. Paternal genetic affinity between Western Austronesians and Daic populations. *BMC Evolutionary Biology* 8: 146.

Pagel, Mark. 2009. Human language as a culturally transmitted replicator. *Genetics* 10: 405–415.

Peyraube, Alain. 2007. Languages and genes in China and in East Asia. *Bulletin of Chinese Linguistics* 2–1: 322–343.

Renfrew, Colin. 1987. *Archeology and Language*. Cambridge: Cambridge University Press.

Ruhlen, Merritt. 1994. *The Origin of Languages. Tracing the Evolution of the Mother Tongue*. New York: Wiley.

Sagart, Laurent, et al. (eds.). 2005. *The peopling of East Asia: Putting together archaeology, linguistics and genetics*. London: Routledge-Curzon.

Schleicher, August. 2009. [1861]. *Compendium der vergleichenden Grammatik der indogermanischen Sprachen*. Cambridge: Cambridge University Press.

Shou, Wei-Hua, and Chun-Jie Xiao. 2010. Y-chromosome distributions among populations in Northwest China identify significant contribution from Central Asian pastoralists and lesser influence of western Eurasians. *Journal of Human Genetics* 55: 314–322.

Strauss, Johann. 2006. Mouvements de convergence et de divergence dans le développement d'un vocabulaire de civilisation des langues islamiques (turc-arabe-persan). In *Contact des Langues II: Les Mots Voyageurs et L'Orient*, ed. M. Bozdémir, and S. Bosnali, 87–127. Istanbul: Presse Universitaire de Boĝaziçi.

Stumpf, Michael P.H., and David B. Goldstein. 2001. Genealogical and evolutionary inference with the human Y chromosome. *Science* 291: 1738–1742.

Underhill, P.A., et al. 2000. Y chromosome sequence variation and the history of human populations. *Nature Genetics* 26: 358–361.

Wang, William. S.-Y. 2000. Linguistic diversity and language relationships. In *New Horizons in Chinese Linguistics*, ed. C.-T. James Huang, and Yen-hui Audrey Li, 235–267. Dordrecht: Kluwer Academic Publishers.

Xu, Dan 2016. Gansu Yongdeng Xuejiawan shaoju diaocha [Investigations on the Xuajiawan language, Yongdeng district, Gansu] *Minzu yuwen* [Non-Han languages] 2, 23–38.

Xu, Dan 2014. *Tangwang hua yanjiu [Studies of the Tangwang language]*. Beijing: Minzu chubanshe.

Xue, Y.L., and C. Tyler-Smith. 2006. Male demography in East Asia: A north-south contrast in human population expansion times. *Genetics* 172: 2431–2439.

Zhou, Ruixia, and Xiaodong Xie. 2008. Origin and evolution of two Yugur sub-clans in Northwest China: A case study in paternal genetic landscape. *Annals of Human Biology* 35 (2): 198–211.

Correlation Between Genetic Structure and Linguistic Phylogeny in East Asia

Yunzhi Huang and Hui Li

Abbreviations

NRY	Non-recombining portion of the Y chromosome
bp	base pairs
mtDNA	mitochondrial DNA
SNP	Single nucleotide polymorphism
STR	Short tandem repeat

1 Introduction

East Asia is a quite separated region from the other parts of the world, with a vast landscape and diverse environments. The climate of East Asia is also unique as monsoon brings the moisture. That results in the unique physical characters of East Asians. The East Asians, with about 22% of the world population, can cursorily be classified into four physical styles, i.e., the Paleolithic migrants (Oceanians), the Azilian migrants (Negrito), the Neolithic migrants (major East Asians), and the Bronze Age migrants (Europeans). Many populations were mixed by some of these four waves of migrations. Since Neolithic Age, they evolved into several cultural confederates. Subsequently, each confederate might have evolved a linguistic family. Today, there are more than 1500 languages in ten linguistic families (Altaic,

Y. Huang (✉) · H. Li (✉)
MOE Key Laboratory of Contemporary Anthropology, School of Life Sciences, Fudan University, Shanghai 200438, People's Republic of China
e-mail: 13110700024@fudan.edu.cn

H. Li
e-mail: LiHui.Fudan@gmail.com

D. Xu and H. Li (eds.), *Languages and Genes in Northwestern China and Adjacent Regions*, DOI 10.1007/978-981-10-4169-3_2

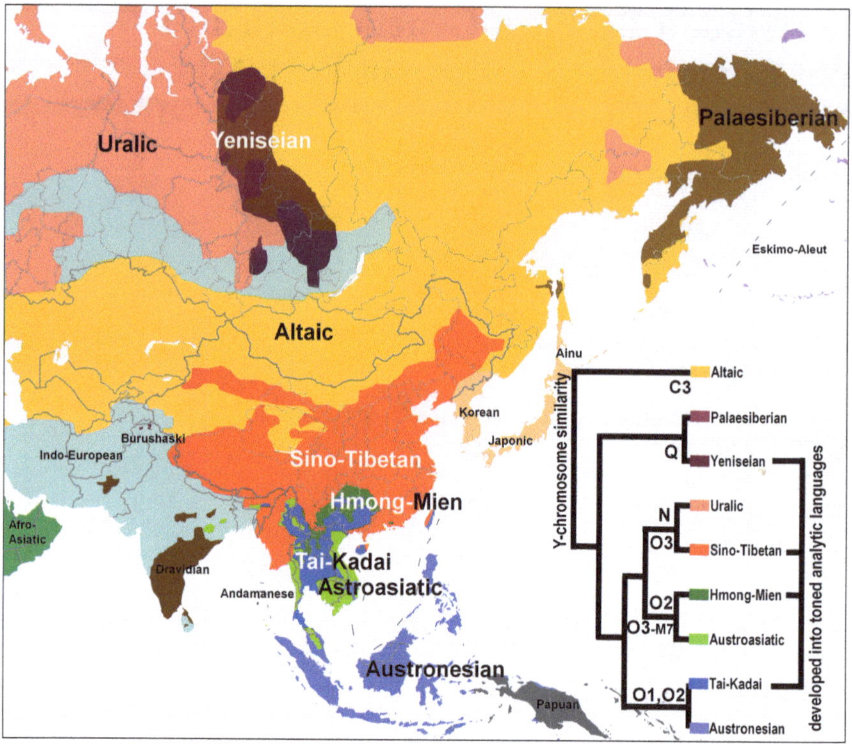

Fig. 1 Distribution of the linguistic families in East Asia and the approximate correlations between languages and Y chromosomes

Austroasiatic, Austronesian, Tai-Kadai, Hmong-Mien, Sino-Tibetan, Uralic, Palaesiberian, Yeniseian, and Indo-European) in East Asia and the flanking regions, which make this region one of the world's most important places for studying human evolution, genetic diversity, and interrelationships between genetics and cultures/languages of human populations (Cavalli-Sforza 1998) (Fig. 1).

2 Correlation Between Autosomal DNA and Linguistic Families

There are three types of genetic materials, i.e., autosomal and X chromosome DNA, paternal Y chromosome, and maternal mitochondrial DNA (mtDNA). Autosomes and X chromosome are inherited from both the parents and are always jumbled by recombination. The non-recombining portion of the Y chromosome (NRY) is strictly inherited paternally, and therefore, is the best material to trace the paternal lineage of the populations with additional advantages of small effective population size, low mutation rate, sufficient markers, and population-specific haplotype distribution (Jobling and Tyler-Smith 1995; Underhill et al. 2000). As the linguistic families were founded in the Neolithic Age, since when people have mostly practiced traditions of patrilocal marriage, the paternal inherited Y chromosomes might be more associated to the linguistic classifications than other genetic materials. However, genetic investigations in the past decade have given more confidence for the relationships between linguistic families and genetic structures in East Asia. The whole genome diversity is also found to be well related to the languages.

Autosomal markers are not always associated to linguistic classifications. When using limited number of markers, the association is usually omitted. However, those markers which have undergone strong selection showed quite good clustering within linguistic families. For example, the *ADH* gene family, which is the most important genes for alcohol metabolism, has been selected for among many East Asian populations (Li et al. 2008a, b). The genetic diversity within *ADH* gene family is associated very well to the linguistic family (Fig. 2), even though only 30 SNP markers were included in the analysis. The Tai-Kadai populations were soundly separated from the Austro-Asiatic populations although they distributed in almost the same geographic region. Not only the genetic diversity, but also the

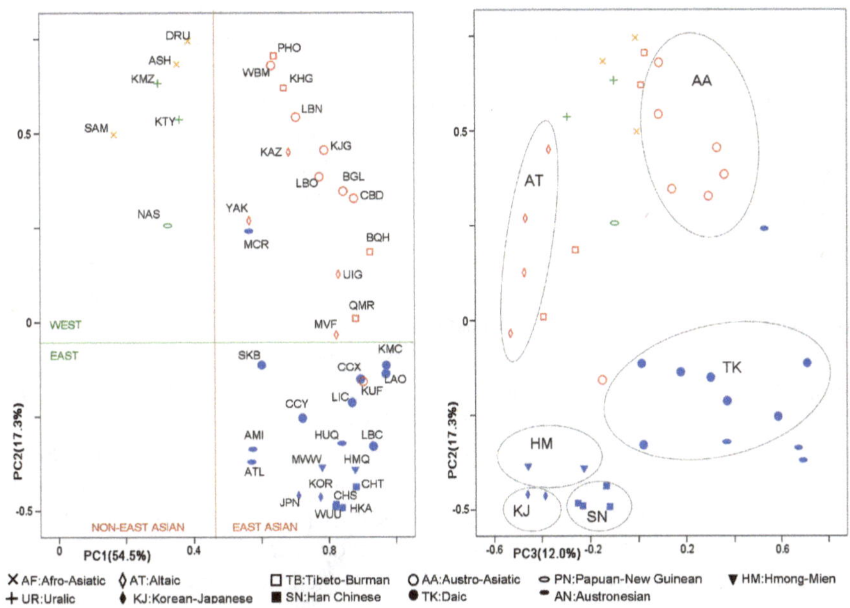

Fig. 2 Principle Analysis Plot based on 30 SNPs within ADH gene family showing clear linguistic clusters

selective signal, was associated with the linguistic families. Strong signals were detected among the Hmong-Mien and Altaic (Korean and Japanese) populations. Week signals were detected among the Han-Chinese populations. And no signal was found in other populations. This association might have resulted from the co-evolution of the *ADH* genes and linguistic families during the Neolithic and Bronze Ages. Further analyses of time estimation suggested that the ADH genes evolved rapidly in East Asia in the recent 5000 years.

When using large number of autosomal polymorphisms, the genetic structure will always be correlated to linguistic families very well among the East Asians. The best sample of such study was carried out by the HUGO Pan-Asian SNP Consortium (2009) since 2005. They analyzed 54,794 autosomal single-nucleotide polymorphisms (SNPs) in 1928 individuals representing 73 Asian and two non-Asian HapMap populations. This large-scale survey of autosomal variation from a broad geographic sample of East Asian human populations showed that genetic ancestry is strongly correlated with linguistic affiliations. Almost all populations from the same linguistic family clustered in the same clade on the genetic phylogeny (Fig. 3). Moreover, the genetic phylogeny showed a geographic association among families. That is, those families distributed in the south were more close to the root, which means that East Asians entered from the south.

The genetic relationships among the linguistic families can be judged from the Structure analysis (genetic components). In this study, 14 components were proved to be the best resolution. The continental populations in East Asia share a common component which can hardly be found in the Southeast Asian Islanders. Specifically, Koreans and Japonic populations share their major component with Sino-Tibetan. Austronesians share their major component with Tai-Kadai populations, which can also be found in Sino-Tibetan populations. Tai-Kadai also comprises a minor component which is major in Austro-Asiatic. Interestingly, the western Austronesians also comprises the Austro-Asiatic major component, while the eastern Austronesians does not. For the Tai-Kadai populations, the closer they reside to the Austro-Asiatic populations, the more Austro-Asiatic components they comprise. This structure suggests that this component originated in Austro-Asiatic populations. Among the Austronesian populations, there are some other exotic components. Those populations in eastern Indonesia where was once the area of Papuans comprise pronounced Papuan components. The Negrito people in Philippines also speak Austronesian while they have their own component besides the Austronesian major component. The Malaysian Negritos have different component from Philippine Negrito as well as a few Austro-Asiatic components. Some small Sino-Tibetan populations migrated to the south have been replaced in genetic components by Austro-Asiatic or Indo-European populations. Altogether, the linguistic families in East Asia show clear association with genetic clusters, and the language contacts are also well recorded by the genetic structure.

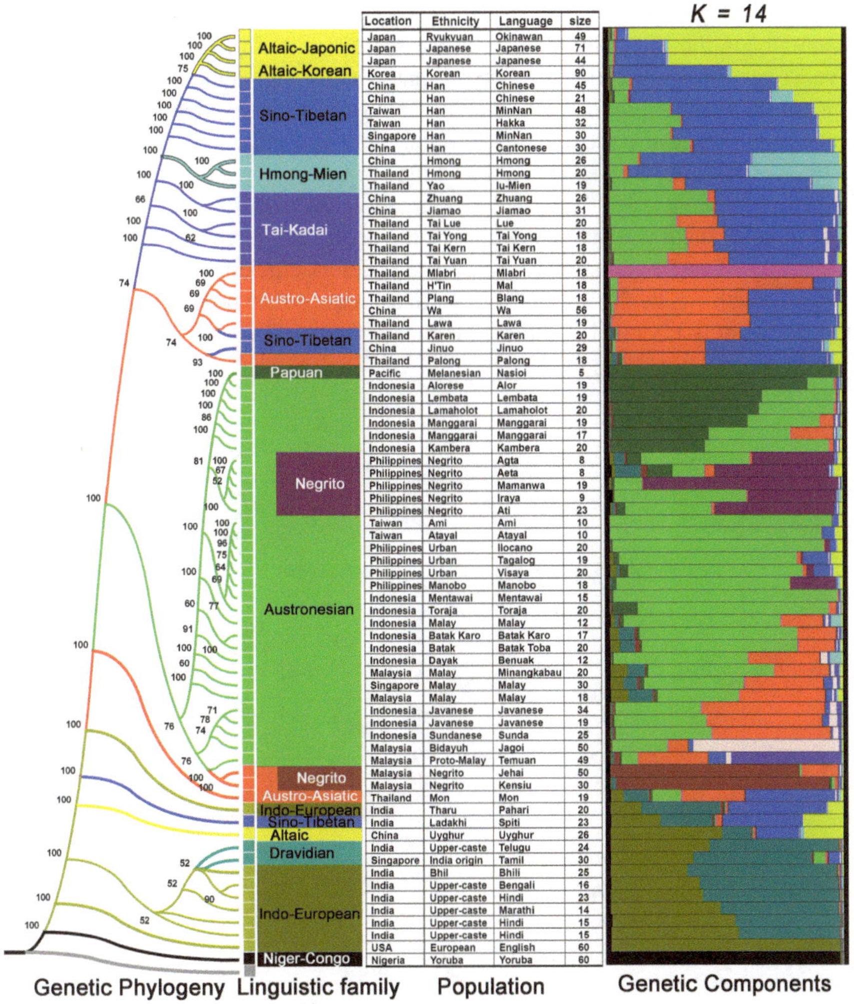

Fig. 3 Genetic structure among the linguistic families in East Asia based on 54,794 autosomal SNPs

3 Mitochondrial DNA or Y Chromosomal DNA

Mitochondrial DNA was first genetic material which came into the success application of molecular anthropology for its advantages of maternal inheritance and large copy number in the cell. The famous "African Eva" hypothesis was just suggested upon global mitochondrial DNA diversity (Cann et al. 1987). It is very clear that mtDNA shows pronounced difference among the geographic regions around world. Those mtDNA haplogroups in Africa are distinctively different from those in western Eurasia. Southern Eurasia and eastern Eurasia also have the unique mtDNA haplogroups. However, mtDNA diversity does not show significant different among the linguistic families in the same region. In East Asia, the mtDNA diversity is clearly correlated to the climate (latitude or altitude). In a principal component analysis plot of East Asian mtDNA, all the arctic populations are in one end and the tropical populations are in the other end (Fig. 4). Populations of the same linguistic family are scattered in different parts of the plot (Qin et al. 2010). Therefore, we concluded that mtDNA is largely influenced by the climate. It is quite easy to understand that mitochondria are the energy resources of cells, and therefore, different mtDNA may have related to different efficiency of energy transformation, which can be the selective stress. In this case, when populations of the same linguistic family migrated to different climates, their mtDNA will changed to adapt

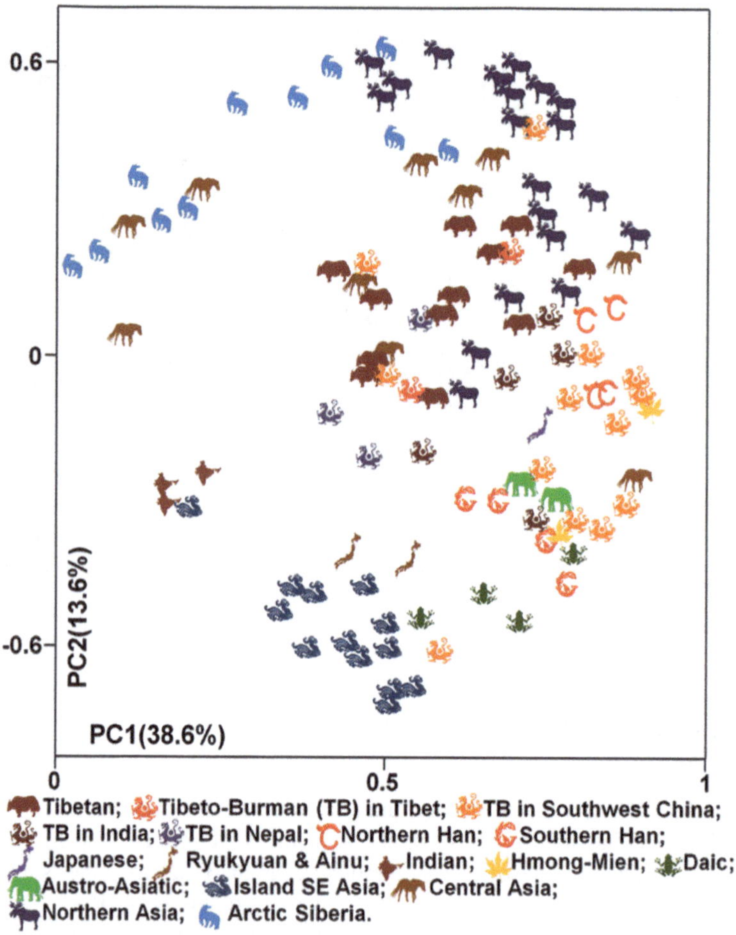

Fig. 4 Principal component analysis plot of the East Asians based on mtDNA diversity

the local climate. Moreover, mtDNA is inherited maternally. Women migrate more frequently between groups by marriages than men in the patrilocal style, which eliminates the possible genetic distance among the linguistic families. Thus, we will not expect the correlation between the linguistic family and mtDNA diversity. Different from mtDNA, the paternal Y chromosome is less frequently transmitted among populations, and therefore, is believed to be more correlated with language.

4 Y Chromosomes Suggested an African Origin for East Asians

Y chromosome studies on East Asians have been widely carried out and have answered many questions about the origin of East Asian populations. For example, the debate on the single or multiple origins of anatomically modern human has lasted for decades. In 1999, Su et al. (1999) used 19 stable and highly informative Y chromosome biallelic markers to assess the genetic structure of the paternal lineages in East Asia, and suggested that modern humans of African descent replaced the previous hominids living in East Asia. In 2001, Ke et al. (2001) examined 12,127 male individuals from 163 populations using three Y chromosome biallelic markers (DE-YAP+, F-M89T, and C-M130T). They found that all the individuals carried a mutation at one of the three sites-YAP, M89, and M130. These three mutations (DE-YAP+, F-M89T, and C-M130T) coalesced to another mutation-M168T (Fig. 5), which originated in Africa at around 64 thousand years ago (Underhill et al. 2000; Ke et al. 2001). Although there have been possible gene flows between archaic hominids and modern humans (Green et al. 2010; Reich et al. 2010; Wang et al. 2013a), it is apparent that the majority of modern human evolved recently in Africa, at least our Y chromosomes all came from Africa. The next question was how the early modern human arrived in East Asia.

Climate has played an important role in human migrations, especially the Last Glacial Period. Last Glacial Period refers to the most recent glacial period from approximately 110 to 10 thousand years ago, covering the Paleolithic and Mesolithic periods of human history (Shi et al. 1989). During this period, when the sea level was much lower than present, many of today's islands were joined to the continents, providing paths for modern human migrations. The maximum extent of glaciation (Last Glacial Maximum, LGM) was between 26.5 and 19–20 thousand years ago, when ice sheets were at their maximum extension and covered much of Asia, northern Europe, and North America (Jobling et al. 2004; Clark et al. 2009). As a consequence, the living space for human was probably very limited in the northern part of Asia. The ice sheets started to recede since 15 thousand years ago and the temperature also began to rise up. This period has really been a flourishing time for modern human migrations.

Here, we focused on the migration histories of East Asian populations achieved by studying Y chromosome and discussed the patterns, and microevolution during

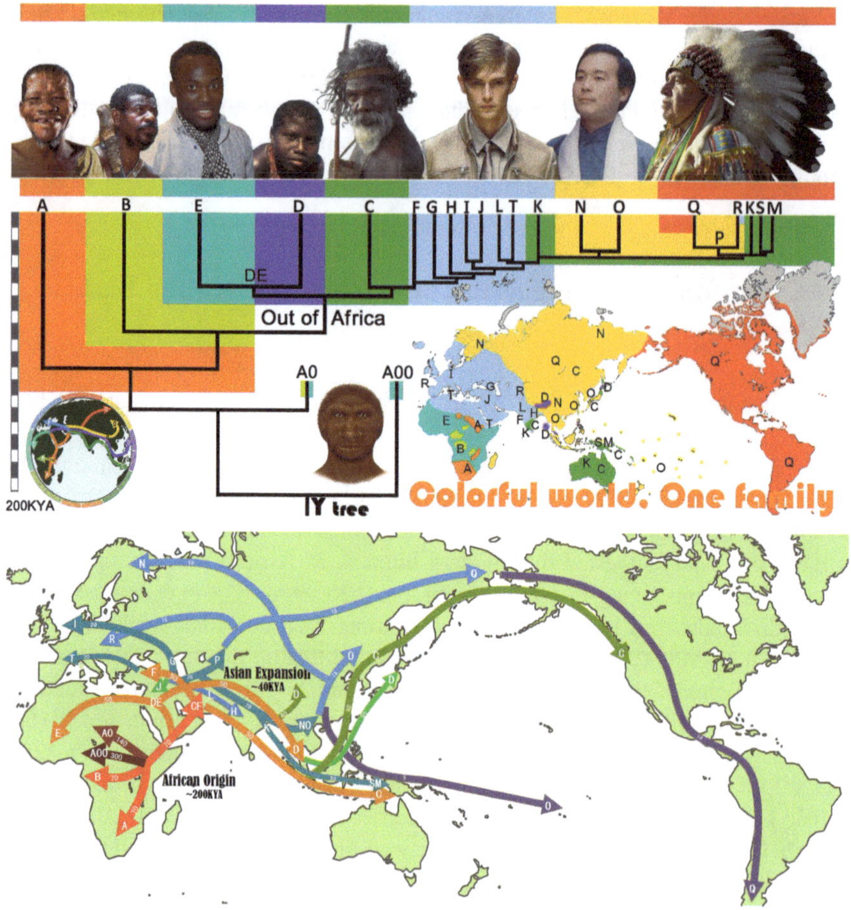

Fig. 5 Y chromosome phylogeny and its migration routes

the initial human settlement and later migrations and expansions in East Asia. It is worthy of note at the very beginning that most time estimations mentioned in this review were achieved using Y chromosome STRs. Although this approach is correct in principle, there is still many ongoing debates about the best way to use STRs in haplogroup dating. In particular, there are two popular used Y chromosome STR mutation rates, i.e., evolutionary rate (Zhivotovsky 2001; Zhivotovsky et al. 2004) and genealogical rate (Gusmão et al. 2005). To choose which mutation rate in the Y chromosome dating is controversial, as the result can be three times different. The high levels of homoplasy and varying mutational properties among loci also largely compromised the accuracy of estimation. Therefore, dates could be only intended as a rough guide for relative haplogroup ages.

5 Northern Route or Southern Route

Once it became generally accepted that modern humans evolved recently in Africa, the times and routes of migration to East Asia remained controversial. Three different models were insisted by different researchers. The first model postulated that northern populations of East Asia migrated to the south, and mixed with the Australian ancestors who had settled in Southeast Asia. The second model suggested that the northern populations of East Asia evolved from the southern settlers. However, a third model assumed that northern and southern East Asian populations have evolved independently since the late Pleistocene more than 10,000 years ago (Jobling et al. 2004; Zhong et al. 2011; Piazza 1998).

There are four dominant Y chromosome macro-haplogroups in East Asia, O-M175, C-M130, D-M174, and N-M231, accounting for about 93% of the East Asian Y chromosomes (Fig. 6). The other haplogroups, such as E-SRY4064,

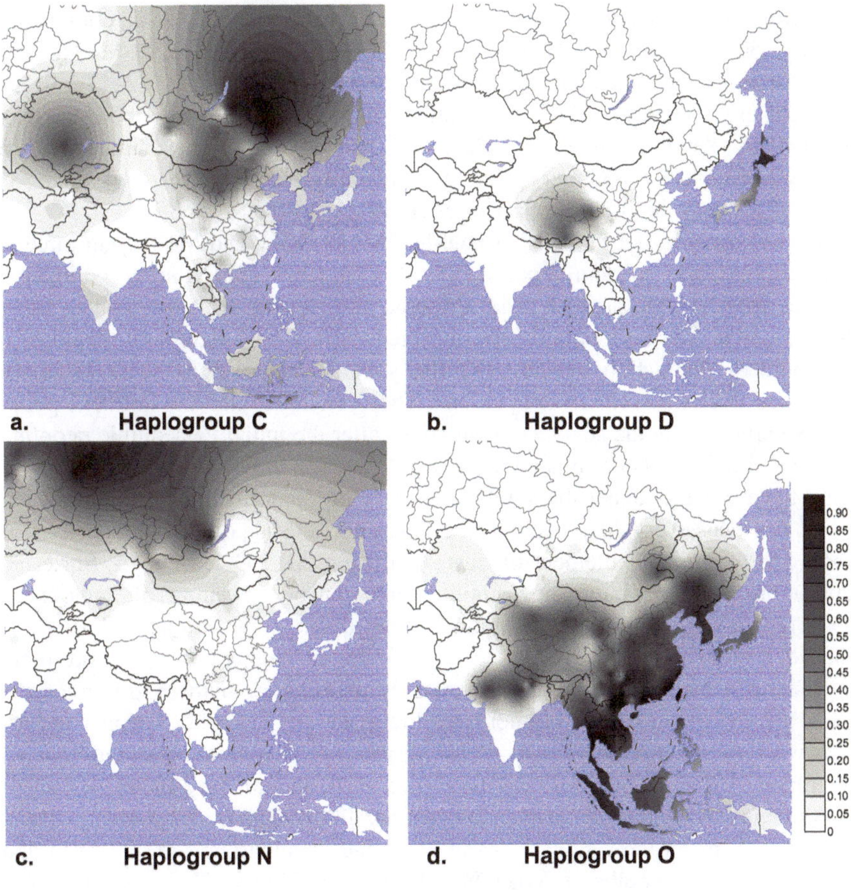

Fig. 6 Geographic distributions of Y chromosome haplogroup C, D, N, and O in East Asia

G-M201, H-M69, I-M170, J-P209, L-M20, Q-M242, R-M207, and T-M70, comprise roughly 7% of the males in East Asia (Zhong et al. 2011).

Haplogroup O-M175 is the largest haplogroup in East Asia, comprising roughly 75% of the Chinese and more than half of the Japanese population and therefore is associated to the Neolithic migrants (Fig. 6). O-M175 gave rise to three downstream haplogroups, O1a-M119, O2-M268, and O3-M122, totaling 60% of the Y chromosomes among East Asian populations (Shi et al. 2005; Yan et al. 2011). Haplogroup O1a-M119 is prevalent along the southeast coast of China, occurring at high frequencies in Tai-Kadai speaking people and Taiwan aborigines (Kayser et al. 2008). O2-M268 accounts for about 5% of the Han Chinese (Yan et al. 2011). O2a1-M95 is the most frequent subclade of O2, which is major haplogroups in the Indo-China Peninsula, and is also found in many populations located in southern China and eastern India (such as Munda) (Kayser et al. 2008; Su et al. 2000). Another subclade of O2, O2b-M176, is most frequent among Koreans and Japanese, and also occurs at very marginal frequencies in Vietnamese and Han Chinese (Ding et al. 2011; Hammer et al. 2006). O3-M122 is the most common haplogroup in China and prevalent throughout East and Southeast Asia, comprising roughly 50–60% of the Han Chinese. O3a1c-002611, O3a2c1-M134, and O3a2c1a-M117 are three main subclades of O3, each accounting for 12–17% of the Han Chinese. O3a2c1a-M117 also exhibits high frequencies in Tibeto-Burman populations. Another subclade O3a2b-M7 reaches the highest frequency in Hmong-Mien and Mon-Khmer speaking populations, but accounts for less than 5% of Han Chinese (Shi et al. 2005; Yan et al. 2011).

Su et al. examined 19 Y-SNPs (including M119, M95, and M122) and three Y chromosome short tandem repeats (STRs) in a large collection of population samples from a wide area of Asia. Principal component analysis of their study showed that all northern populations clustered together and were well included in the southern population cluster, and the southern populations were far more diversified than the northern populations. They concluded that the northern populations derived from the southern populations after the initial Palaeolithic peopling of East Asia. They also estimated the age of O3-M122 to be 18–60 thousand years using three Y-STRs under the single-step mutation model with a mutation rate of 0.18% per locus every 20 years, which might reflect the age of the bottleneck event leading to the initial settlement of East Asia (Su et al. 1999). In 2005, Shi et al. (2005) presented a systematic sampling and genetic screening of haplogroup O3-M122 in more than 2000 individuals from diverse populations in East Asia. Their data showed that the O3-M122 haplogroups in southern East Asia are more diverse than those in northern East Asia, supporting a southern origin of the O3-M122. The time of the early northward migration of O3-M122 lineages in East Asia was estimated about 25–30 thousand years ago using the average squared difference (ASD) method with an average Y-STR evolutionary mutation rate of 0.00069 per locus per 25 years (Zhivotovsky 2001; Zhivotovsky et al. 2004). Recently, Cai et al. (2011) examined the haplogroup O3a2b-M7 and O3a2c1a-M117 in Southeast Asian Mon-Khmer and Hmong-Mien speaking populations, and indicated a unidirectional diffusion through bottlenecks from

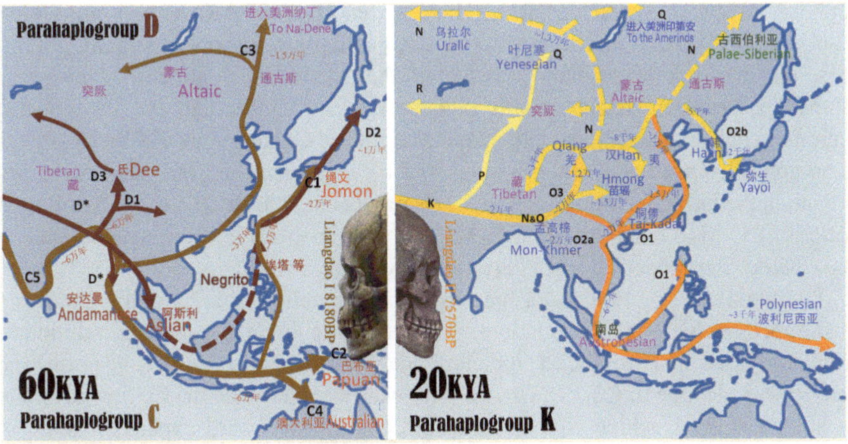

Fig. 7 Migration of the Y chromosome haplogroup C, D, N, and O in East Asia. Broken lines represent for alternative migration routes

Southeast Asia into East Asia about 19,000 years ago (also using the ASD method with an average Y-STR evolutionary mutation rate of 0.00069 per locus per 25 years) during the Last Glacial Maximum. A general south-to-north Y-STR diversity decline was also observed in haplogroup O3a1c-002611, suggesting that haplogroup O3a1c also migrated northward along with other O3-M122 lineages (Wang et al. 2013b). Therefore, the southern route of the early human migration in East Asia, taking the largest Y haplogroups O, is supported by most evidences (Fig. 7).

6 Earliest Settlement in East Asia

The age of haplogroup O in East Asia is no more than 30 thousand years when estimated from sufficient numbers (>7) of STR markers. Therefore, haplogroup O was not the earliest Y chromosome carried by modern human into East Asia. Haplogroup C-M130 may represent one of the earliest settlements in East Asia. Haplogroup C has a high to moderate frequency in Far East and Oceania, and lower frequency in Europe and the Americas, but is absent in Africa (Fig. 6). Several geographically specific subclades of haplogroup C have been identified, i.e., C1-M8, C2-M38, C3-M217, C4-M347, C5-M356, and C6-P55 (Zhong et al. 2010). Haplogroup C3-M217 is the most widespread subclade, and reaches the highest frequencies among the populations of Mongolia and Siberia. Haplogroup C1-M8 is absolutely restricted to the Japanese and Ryukyuans, appearing at a low frequency of about 5% or less. Haplogroup C2-M38 is found among certain local populations on Pacific Islands from eastern Indonesia to Polynesia. Especially among the populations of Polynesia, C2 has become the modal haplogroup due to severe founder effects and genetic drift (Hammer et al. 2006; Kayser et al. 2006). Haplogroup C4-M347 is the most common haplogroup among Australian aborigines, and has not been found outside of the Australian continent. Haplogroup C5-M356 has been detected with low frequency in India and the neighboring regions in Pakistan and Nepal (Sengupta et al. 2006; Gayden et al. 2007). C6-P55 is geographically restricted to the highland of New Guinea (P55 has been moved to private in the latest Y chromosome tree) (Karafet et al. 2008). This wide distribution pattern of C-M130 suggests that C-M130 might arise somewhere in mainland of Asia before the modern humans arrived in Southeast Asia.

To give a clear picture about the origin and migration of haplogroup C, Zhong et al. typed twelve Y-SNPs and eight Y-STRs among 465 haplogroup C individuals from 140 East and Southeast Asian populations. A general south-to-north and east-to-west decline of C3 Y-STR diversity was observed with the highest diversity in Southeast Asia, which supports a single coastal northward expansion route of haplogroup C3 in China about 32–42 thousand years ago using the ASD method with an average Y-STR evolutionary mutation rate of 0.00069 per locus per 25 years (Zhong et al. 2010) (Fig. 7). The arrival of haplogroup C in Southeast Asia and Australia must be much earlier than that time at around 60 thousand years ago. Therefore, populations with haplogroup C must have settled in East Asia some ten thousand years earlier than those with haplogroup O.

7 Genetic Legacy of the Paleolithic Period

The migration history of haplogroup D-M174 is most mysterious. By the time, we have known little about the origin and dispersal of this haplogroup. This haplogroup was derived from African haplogroup DE-M1 (YAP insertion) and is associated with a short black Asian physical style. Haplogroups E and D are brother haplogroups. While haplogroup E was carried westwards to the Africa by the tall black people, haplogroup D might have carried eastwards to East Asia by the short black people (Fig. 5).

Haplogroup D-M174 has high frequencies in the Andaman Negritos, the northern Tibeto-Burman populations, and the Ainu of Japan, and also appears at low frequencies in other East and Southeast Asian and Central Asian populations (Fig. 6) (Su et al. 2000; Hammer et al. 2006; Karafet et al. 2001; Thangaraj et al. 2003). A northern Tibeto-Burman population, the Baima-Dee, comprises nearly 100% of haplogroup D. There are three main subclades of haplogroup D, i.e., D1-M15, D2-M55, and D3-P99, and many unclassified minor sub-haplogroups. Haplogroup D1-M15 is prevalent in the Tibetans, Tangut-Chiang, and Lolo, and also found at very low frequencies among the mainland East Asian populations (Shi et al. 2008; Wen et al. 2004a, b). Haplogroup D2-M55 is restricted to various populations of the Japanese Archipelago. Haplogroup D3-P99 is found at high frequencies among Tibetans and several Tibeto-Burman minorities in Sichuan and Yunnan provinces that reside in close proximity to the Tibetans, such as Pumi and Naxi (Shi et al.

2008). The paragroup D* is restricted to Andaman Islands (Thangaraj et al. 2003), which has been isolated for at least 20 thousand years. Some other minor haplogroups, also included in D*, can be found around Tibet. Most of the populations with haplogroup D have very dark skin color, including the Andamanese, some of the Tibeto-Burman and Mon-Khmer people. The Ainu people may have changed to pale skin to absorb more ultraviolet light in high latitude region.

For the origin of haplogroup D, Chandrasekar et al. (2007) suggested that the CT-M168 gave rise to the YAP insertion and D-M174 mutation in South Asia based their findings of the YAP insertion in northeast Indian tribes and the D-M174 in Andaman islanders. In that case, haplogroup E with YAP insertion might also have an Asian origin. However, this hypothesis is seldom supported by any evidence. If haplogroup D originated in Africa, it is most mysterious how it has traveled through the populations with haplogroups CF to East Asia.

Another mystery is how haplogroup D has migrated from southwest of East Asia all the way to Japan. It could have gone either through mainland East Asian or through Sundaland (Fig. 7). The mainland route seems to be shorter than the Sundaland route. Shi et al. proposed that the northward expansion of D-M174 to western China might predate the migrations of other major East Asian lineages at about 60 thousand years ago using ASD time estimation method with an average Y-STR evolutionary mutation rate of 0.00069 per locus per 25 years. Subsequently, these frontier populations could have traveled eastwards through a northern route via Korea or through a southern route via Taiwan and Ryukyu land bridge to Japan, where they might meet the earlier Australian style settlers. The current relic D-M174 in East Asia was probably edged out of eastern China by the later northward migration of haplogroup O and the Neolithic expansion of Han Chinese (Shi et al. 2008). However, there has never been any evidence from genetics or archaeology that haplogroup D2 or Negritos have migrated to eastern China. In contrast, there are still many Negrito populations in Sundaland from Malaya to the Philippines. It was possible that Negritos have occupied the whole Sundaland in late Paleolithic Age. Therefore, these populations might move directly from the Philippines to Taiwan and Ryukyu. The only problem is that no haplogroup D has been found in the Negritos in the Philippines. Their paternal lineages might have been replaced by the expansion of haplogroups C2 and K from Papua around 18 thousand years ago using BATWING time estimation method (Delfin et al. 2011) or much recent migration of haplogroup O from mainland East Asia (Scholes et al. 2011). However, due to the lack of data, the history of haplogroup D, as a genetic legacy of Azilian Age in East Asia, remains mysterious.

8 Recent Immigrations of Uralic and Altaic Populations

Haplogroup O has a brother haplogroup, N-M231, which reaches highest frequency in northern Eurasia, especially among most of the Uralic populations, including Finnic, Ugric, Samoyedic, and Yukaghir people, as well as some Altaic and Eskimo populations in northern Siberia. It also appears at a low frequency in East Asia (Fig. 6) (Karafet et al. 2001; Rootsi et al. 2007). Detailed analysis of haplogroup N suggested a more recent expansion on a counter-clock northern route from inner East Asia or southern Siberia about 12–14 thousand years ago using ASD time estimation method with an average Y-STR evolutionary mutation rate of 0.00069 per locus per 25 years, which explained high frequency of haplogroup N in northeast Europe (Rootsi et al. 2007). Subclade N1a-M128 is found at low frequency among populations in northern China, such as Manchu, Xibe, Evenks, Korean, and also among some Turkic populations in Central Asia. Haplogroup N1b-P43 is approximately 6–8 thousand years old using ASD time estimation method with an average Y-STR evolutionary mutation rate of 0.00069 per locus per 25 years and probably originated in Siberia. N1b is prevalent in the Northern Samoyeds, and also occurs at low to moderate frequencies among some other Uralic and Altaic peoples (Derenko et al. 2007; Mirabal et al. 2009). The most frequent subclade N1c-Tat arose probably in China around 14 thousand years ago (ASD method with a mutation rate of 0.00069 per locus per 25 years) and subsequently experienced a serial of founder effects or strong bottlenecks in Siberia and a secondary expansion in East Europe (Rootsi et al. 2007). These studies traced the origin of haplogroup N to southwestern China and Southeast Asia. Our recent studies revealed that haplogroup N reaches the pronounced high diversity in Han Chinese populations, which suggested a Han Chinese origin of haplogroup N. Those proportions in North Asia and Southeast Asia are two distinctive clades out of Han Chinese. In this case, most paternal lineages of Uralic speakers originated in the ancestors of Han Chinese.

The migration of haplogroup N is another evidence for the southern origin of the East Asians. However, there were still studies against the southern origin of East Asians. Karafet et al. examined 52 Y-SNPs in 1383 individuals of 25 populations from East Asia and Central Asia. They found the average pairwise difference among haplogroups was noticeably smaller in southern East Asia and there was no genetic divergence between southern and northern East Asia (Karafet et al. 2001). Xue et al. (2009) applied a Bayesian full-likelihood analysis to 45 Y-SNPs and 16 Y-STRs data from 988 men of 27 populations from China, Mongolia, Korea, and Japan. They reported the Y-STRs have a higher diversity in northern East Asian populations than that in southern populations. The northern populations expanded earlier than the southern populations. However, Shi et al. (2008) pointed out that the larger diversity among Y-chromosome haplogroups observed in northern East Asia claimed by Karafet et al. (2001) is actually a false impression due to recent population admixture. The study of Xue et al. (2009) has the similar drawback. The high gene diversity observed in Mongols, Uighurs, and Manchurians was probably due to their recent extensive admixture with Central Asian, West Eurasian, and Han Chinese populations. Furthermore, the southern populations studied by Xue et al. were not sufficient and the within-population bottleneck effect caused by long-time geographic isolation might have a great impact on gene diversity estimation.

The subsequent debate focuses on how to interpret the Central Asia and West Eurasia related genetic components in East Asia. Zhong et al. (2011) sampled 3,826 males from 117 populations and performed high-resolution genotyping to address this problem. In the study of Zhong et al. haplogroups O-M175, C-M130, D-M174, and N-M231 still suggest the substantial contribution of the southern route. However, the Central Asia and West Eurasia related haplogroups, such as haplogroups R-M207 and Q-M242, occur primarily in northwestern East Asia and their frequencies gradually decrease from west to east. In addition, the Y-STR diversities of haplogroups R-M207 and Q-M242 also indicate the existence of northern route migration about 18,000 years ago (ASD method with a mutation rate of 0.00069 per locus per 25 years) from Central Asia to North Asia, and recent population admixture along the Silk Road since about 3000 years ago (Piazza 1998).

The current populations speaking the languages within the Altaic family show great genetic incoherence. Although Mongolic and Tungus speakers are similar with high frequencies of haplogroup C, Turkic speakers are not the same but admixed populations with various genetic components. Haplogroup R, C, N, Q, O, J, etc. can all be detected in Turkic speaking populations with fluctuant frequencies (Fig. 8). Therefore, genetic evidences do not support the affiliation of Turkic in Altaic family. We neither found any evidence supporting the Xiongnu ancestral for Turkic or Mongol-Tungus populations. Most of the Y haplogroups of the ancient Xiongnu samples are Q (Huang and Li 2015), while few haplogroup Q can be found in the present Turkic or Mongol-Tungus populations. On another hand, high frequencies of haplogroup Q were found among the Yeniseian and Palaesiberian speaking populations, suggesting that these two families are more likely closely related to Xiongnu in paternal lineages.

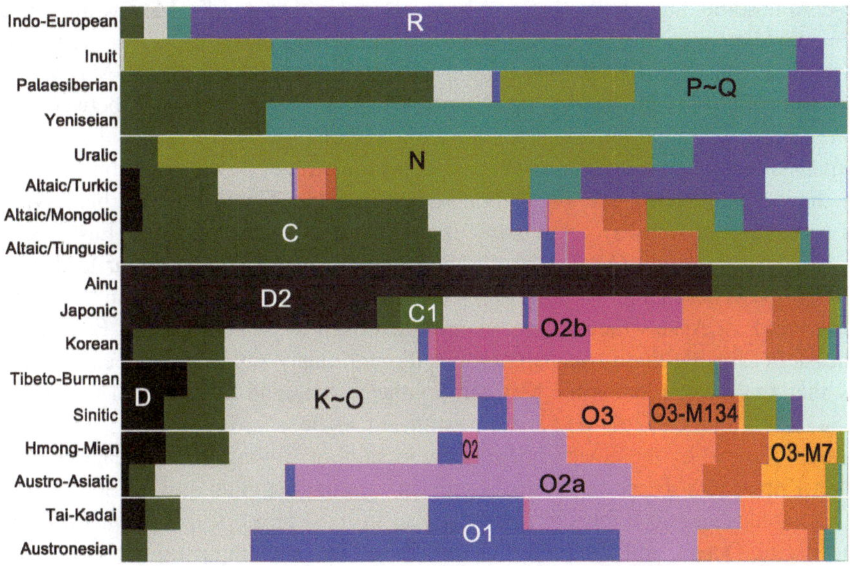

Fig. 8 Y chromosome haplogroup frequencies of the East Asian populations speaking languages of certain families

9 Genetic Coherences for Linguistic Families

The genetic patterns in human societies are often influenced by their cultural practices, such as residence patterns and subsistence strategies. Y chromosomes of East Asian populations have played an important role in documenting such influences, e.g., relationships among patrilocal populations should have stronger association with Y chromosomes than with mtDNA. East Asian languages show strong association with paternal lineages of Y chromosomes (Shi et al. 2005; Cai et al. 2011; Zhong et al. 2010; Wen et al. 2004a; Kumar et al. 2007) and whole genomic diversity (The HUGO Pan-Asian SNP Consortium 2009), but not maternal lineages of mtDNA. Y chromosome haplogroup O3-M134 is associated with Sino-Tibetan speakers (Shi et al. 2005; Wen et al. 2004a); O2-M95 is with Austro-Asiatic speakers (Kumar et al. 2007). Moreover, phylogenetic structure among the linguistic families suggested by the linguistics is also supported by Y chromosomes but not by whole genomic diversity, e.g., linguistic affinity between Hmong-Mien and Austro-Asiatic languages was proved by Y chromosome marker O3-M7 (Cai et al. 2011); and that between Tai-Kadai and Austronesian languages by O1-M119 (Li et al. 2008a, b).

Most of the Y-chromosome lineages of East Asians came from Southeast Asia. In that case, the indigenous populations of Southeast Asia, Austro-Asiatic (Mon-Khmer), should be the oldest population in East Asia. However, very few Mon-Khmer populations had been investigated, and therefore, little was known about the purported migrations from Southeast Asia into East Asia and their roles in shaping the genetic structure of East Asian populations. We analyzed the Y-chromosome data from 1652 individuals belonging to 47 Mon-Khmer and Hmong-Mien speaking populations that are distributed primarily across Southeast Asia and extend into East Asia (Cai et al. 2011). Haplogroup O3a3b-M7, which appears mainly in Mon-Khmer and Hmong-Mien, indicates a strong tie between the two groups. The short tandem repeat network of O3a3b-M7 displayed a hierarchical expansion structure (annual ring shape), with Mon-Khmer haplotypes being located at the original point, and the Hmong-Mien and the Tibeto-Burman haplotypes distributed further away from core of the network. Moreover, the East Asian dominant haplogroup O3a3c1-M117 shows a network structure similar to that of O3a3b-M7. These patterns indicate an early unidirectional diffusion from Southeast Asia into East Asia, which might have resulted from the genetic drift of East Asian ancestors carrying these two haplogroups through many small bottle-necks formed by the complicated landscape between Southeast Asia and East Asia. The ages of O3a3b-M7 and O3a3c1-M117 were estimated to be approximately 19 thousand years, followed by the emergence of the ancestors of Hmong-Mien lineages out of Mon-Khmer and the unidirectional northward migrations into East Asia.

Austronesian is a linguistic family spread in most areas of the Southeast Asia, the Pacific Ocean, and the Indian Ocean. Based on their linguistic similarity, this linguistic family included Malayo-Polynesians and Taiwan aborigines. The linguistic similarity also led to the controversial hypothesis that Taiwan is the homeland of all the Malayo-Polynesians, a hypothesis that has been debated by ethnologists, linguists, archaeologists, and geneticists. It is well accepted that the Eastern Austronesians (Micronesians and Polynesians) derived from the Western Austronesians (Island Southeast Asians and Taiwanese), and that the Tai-Kadai populations on the mainland are supposed to be the headstream of all the Austronesian populations. To assess the relationships between the three ethnic groups, we studied 20 SNPs and 7 STRs in the non-recombining region of the 1509 Y chromosomes from 30 China Tai-Kadai populations, 23 Indonesian and Vietnam Malayo-Polynesian populations, and 11 Taiwan aboriginal populations (Li et al. 2008a, b). These three groups show many resemblances in paternal lineages. Admixture analyses demonstrated that the Tai-Kadai populations are hardly influenced by Han Chinese genetically, and that they make up the largest proportion of Indonesians. Most of the population samples contain a high frequency of haplogroup O1a-M119, which is nearly absent in other ethnic families. The STR network of haplogroup O1a* illustrated that Indonesian lineages did not derive from Taiwan aborigines as linguistic studies suggest, but from Tai-Kadai populations. We show that, in contrast to the Taiwan homeland hypothesis, the Island Southeast Asians do not have a Taiwan origin based on their paternal lineages. Furthermore, we show that both Taiwan aborigines and Indonesians likely derived from the Tai-Kadai populations based on their paternal lineages. These two populations seem to have evolved independently of each other. Our results indicate that a super-phylum, which includes Taiwan aborigines, Tai-Kadai, and Malayo-Polynesians, is genetically educible.

The Sino-Tibetan populations comprise the major population of East Asia. The geographic distribution of this group is very vast. Judging from languages and physical features, both subgroups, Han Chinese and Tibeto-Burman, exhibit pronounced differences between north and south. It has been argued whether southern Han and northern Han have the same origin and in turn the same genetic pattern. The same question was also existed for Tibeto-Burman. The spread of culture and language in human populations is explained by two alternative models: the demic diffusion model, which involves mass movement of people; and the cultural diffusion model, which refers to cultural impact between populations and involves limited genetic exchange between them. The mechanism of the peopling of Europe has long been debated, a key issue being whether the diffusion of agriculture and language from the Near East was concomitant with a large movement of farmers. By systematically analysing Y-chromosome and mitochondrial DNA variation in Han populations, we found that the pattern of the southward expansion of Han culture is consistent with the demic diffusion model, and that males played a larger role than females in this expansion (Wen et al. 2004a) (Fig. 9).

Among the ten Chinese linguistic branches, the Pinghua branch in Guangxi is genetically different. We have studied eight Pinghua populations and other ethnic groups (Zhuang, Kam, Mulam, Laka, and Mien) from Guangxi Zhuang Autonomous Region of China. Both mtDNA and the Y chromosomes were typed in these samples (Gan et al. 2008; Lu et al. 2013). High frequencies of the Y chromosome haplogroups O2a* and O*, which always present at a high frequency

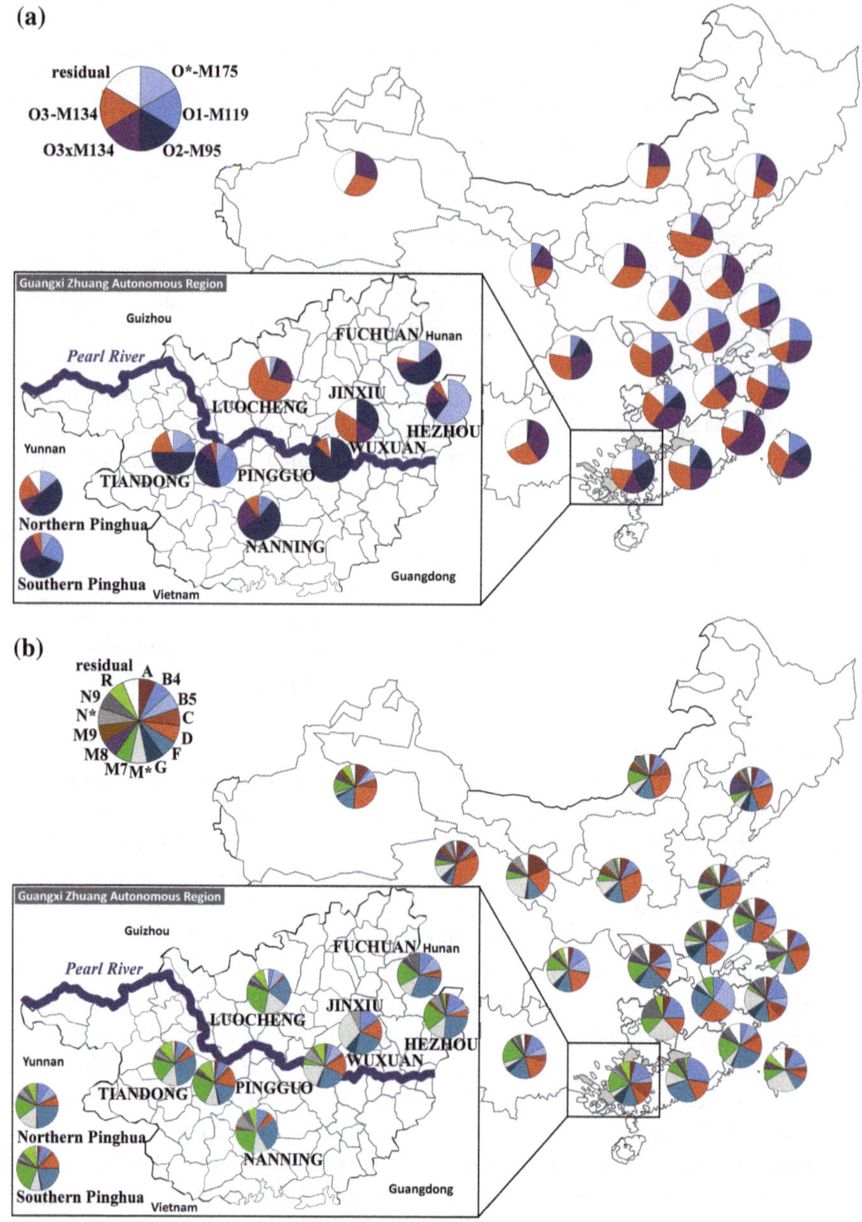

Fig. 9 Y chromosomal and mitochondrial diversity shows that Pinghua is an exception of the genetic coherence of Han Chinese

among the populations of the southern minorities, were found in Pinghua populations. Only Pinghua populations in Luocheng and Jinxiu maintain the Han frequent haplogroup O3a5a. MtDNA lineages B4a, B5a, M*, F1a, M7b1, and N* were found in Pinghua populations, exhibiting a pattern similar to the neighboring indigenous populations, especially the Tai-Kadai populations. Cluster analyses of Pinghua populations, the other Han branches, and other ethnic groups in East Asia indicated that Pinghua populations are much closer to the southern minorities than to the other Han branches. Admixture analyses confirmed this result. Therefore, we argue that Pinghua populations did not descend from Han Chinese, but from southern minorities. The ancestral populations of Pinghua people were assimilated by the Han Chinese in terms of language, culture, and self-identification and, consequently, the Pinghua people became an exceptional branch of Han Chinese's coherent genetic structure.

Tibeto-Burman populations were historically derived from ancient tribes of northwestern China and subsequently moved to the south, where they admixed with the southern natives during the past 2600 years. They are currently extensively distributed in China and Southeast Asia. We analyze the variations of 965 Y chromosomes and 754 mtDNAs in >20 Tibeto-Burman populations from China (Wen et al. 2004b). By examining the haplotype group distributions of Y-chromosome and mtDNA markers and their principal components, we show that the genetic structure of the extant southern Tibeto-Burman populations were primarily formed by two parental groups: northern immigrants and native southerners. Furthermore, the admixture has a bias between male and female lineages, with a stronger influence of northern immigrants on the male lineages (approximately 62%) and with the southern natives contributing more extensively to the female lineages (approximately 56%) in the extant southern Tibeto-Burman populations. This is the first genetic evidence revealing sex-biased admixture in southern Tibeto-Burman populations, which has genetic, historical, and anthropological implications.

The association between languages and Y chromosomes but not mtDNA might reflect sex-bias migrations due to patrilocality. Patrilocality refers to the social system that a married couple resides with or near the husband's parents. Forster et al. suggested that it may often be the language of the father that is dominant within the family group if the parents have different linguistic backgrounds (Forster and Renfrew 2011). However, as the whole genomic diversity is also associated with linguistic families, both paternal and maternal lineages must have been well kept since the linguistic families emerged. Therefore, the loss of association between mtDNA and languages might not simply be explained by a social nature of women adoption. There might be a higher effective population size in ancient population for females than for males due to frequent hunting activities and wars, and thus, the original mtDNA variation of a language group was less affected by genetic drift. Other interpretations might also be possible, such as preferential males, the number of offspring, and the different mutation rates, etc.

10 Conclusions and Perspectives

Y chromosome plays an important role in unraveling the entangled history of modern human populations in East Asia. Although many questions remain unresolved, a clear framework of the prehistory has been obtained. Four Y chromosome haplogroups C, D, O, and N, accounted for more than 90% of the East Asian Y chromosomes, are suggested to have Southeast Asian origins, carried by three waves of migrations. The distributions of western Eurasia specific Y chromosome haplogroups E, G, H, I, J, L, Q, R, and T in northwest China reflect the recent gene flows from the west and the probable northern route migration. A west-to-east decline of these western haplogroups was clearly observed. Linguistic families are well associated with the Y chromosome diversity.

However, current Y chromosome researches in East Asia are limited in two important aspects. The first limit is the poor resolution for those East Asian specific Y chromosome branches, such as haplogroup O-M175. Despite the huge population of haplogroup O, there have been much less markers defined in haplogroup O than in haplogroups R and E. For instance, three Y-SNP markers, 002611, M134, and M117, represent about 260 million people in East Asia, but downstream markers are far from enough to reveal informative genetic substructures of those populations. The second limit is inaccurate estimation of lineage and population divergence time as mentioned at the beginning.

The advent of next-generation sequencing technology made it possible to sequence the entire Y chromosome in numerous human individuals and in deep-rooting pedigrees. For instance, The 1000 Genomes Project Consortium has already sequenced the Y chromosomes at an average depth of 1.83 in 77 males in the low-coverage project, and 15.23 depth in the two trio fathers (1000 Genomes Project Consortium 2010). Further deep sequencing will offer a solution for both enhanced Y chromosome phylogenetic resolution and accurate calibration of the molecular clock in evolutionary studies.

Acknowledgements This work was supported by the National Excellent Youth Science Foundation of China (31222030) and Shanghai Rising-Star Program (12QA1400300).

References

1000 Genomes Project Consortium. 2010. A map of human genome variation from population-scale sequencing. *Nature* 467: 1061–1073.

Cai, X., Z. Qin, B. Wen, S. Xu, Y. Wang, Y. Lu, L. Wei, C. Wang, S. Li, X. Huang, L. Jin, and H. Li. 2011. Genographic Consortium: Human migration through bottlenecks from Southeast Asia into East Asia during last glacial maximum revealed by Y chromosomes. *PLoS ONE* 6 (8): e24282.

Cann, R.L., M. Stoneking, and A.C. Wilson. 1987. Mitochondrial DNA and human evolution. *Nature* 325 (6099): 31–36.

Cavalli-Sforza, L.L. 1998. The Chinese human genome diversity project. *Proceedings of the National Academy of Sciences of the United States of America* 95: 11501–11503.

Chandrasekar, A., S.Y. Saheb, P. Gangopadyaya, S. Gangopadyaya, A. Mukherjee, D. Basu, G.R. Lakshmi, A.K. Sahani, B. Das, S. Battacharya, S. Kumar, D. Xaviour, D. Sun, and V.R. Rao. 2007. YAP insertion signature in South Asia. *Annals of Human Biology* 34: 582–586.

Clark, P.U., A.S. Dyke, J.D. Shakun, A.E. Carlson, J. Clark, B. Wohlfarth, J.X. Mitrovica, S.W. Hostetler, and A.M. McCabe. 2009. The last glacial maximum. *Science* 325: 710–714.

Delfin, F., J.M. Salvador, G.C. Calacal, H.B. Perdigon, K.A. Tabbada, L.P. Villamor, S.C. Halos, E. Gunnarsdóttir, S. Myles, D.A. Hughes, S. Xu, L. Jin, O. Lao, M. Kayser, M.E. Hurles, M. Stoneking, and M.C. De Ungria. 2011. The Y-chromosome landscape of the Philippines: Extensive heterogeneity and varying genetic affinities of Negrito and non-Negrito groups. *European Journal of Human Genetics* 19: 224–230.

Derenko, M., B. Malyarchuk, G. Denisova, M. Wozniak, T. Grzybowski, I. Dambueva, and I. Zakharov. 2007. Y-chromosome haplogroup N dispersals from south Siberia to Europe. *Journal of Human Genetics* 52 (9): 763–770.

Ding, Q.L., C.C. Wang, S.E. Farina, and H. Li. 2011. Mapping human genetic diversity on the Japanese archipelago. *Advances in Anthropology* 1 (2): 19–25.

Forster, P., and C. Renfrew. 2011. Mother tongue and Y chromosomes. *Science* 333: 1390–1391.

Gan, R.J., S.L. Pan, L.F. Mustavich, Z.D. Qin, X.Y. Cai, J. Qian, C.W. Liu, J.H. Peng, S.L. Li, J.S. Xu, L. Jin, and H. Li. 2008. Genographic Consortium: Pinghua population as an exception of Han Chinese's coherent genetic structure. *Journal of Human Genetics* 53: 303–313.

Gayden, T., A.M. Cadenas, M. Regueiro, N.B. Singh, L.A. Zhivotovsky, P.A. Underhill, L.L. Cavalli-Sforza, and R.J. Herrera. 2007. The Himalayas as a directional barrier to gene flow. *American Journal of Human Genetics* 80: 884–894.

Green, R.E., J. Krause, A.W. Briggs, T. Maricic, U. Stenzel, M. Kircher, Nick Patterson, H. Li, W. W. Zhai, M.H.Y. Fritz, N.F. Hansen, E.Y. Durand, A.S. Malaspinas, J.D. Jensen, T. Marques-Bonet, C. Alkan, Kay Prüfer, M. Meyer, H.A. Burbano, J.M. Good, R. Schultz, A. Aximu-Petri, A. Butthof, B. Hber, B. Hffner, M. Siegemund, A. Weihmann, C. Nusbaum, E.S. Lander, C. Russ, N. Novod, J. Affourtit, M. Egholm, C. Verna, P. Rudan, Dejana Brajkovic, Ž. Kucan, I. Gušic, V.B. Doronichev, L.V. Golovanova, C. Lalueza-Fox, M. Rasilla, J. Fortea, A. Rosas, R.W. Schmitz, P.L.F. Johnson, E.E. Eichler, D. Falush, E. Birney, J.C. Mullikin, M. Slatkin, R. Nielsen, J. Kelso, M. Lachmann, D. Reich, and S. Pääbo. 2010. A draft sequence of the Neandertal genome. *Science* 328: 710–722.

Gusmão, L., P. Sánchez-Diz, F. Calafell, P. Martín, C.A. Alonso, F. Alvarez-Fernández, C. Alves, L. Borjas-Fajardo, W.R. Bozzo, M.L. Bravo, J.J. Builes, J. Capilla, M. Carvalho, C. Castillo, C.I. Catanesi, D. Corach, Lonardo A.M. Di, R. Espinheira, E. Fagundes de Carvalho, M. J. Farfán, H.P. Figueiredo, I. Gomes, M.M. Lojo, M. Marino, M.F. Pinheiro, M.L. Pontes, V. Prieto, E. Ramos-Luis, J.A. Riancho, A.C. Souza Góes, O.A. Santapa, D.R. Sumita, G. Vallejo, L. Vidal Rioja, M.C. Vide, C.I. Vieira da Silva, M.R. Whittle, W. Zabala, M.T. Zarrabeitia, A. Alonso, A. Carracedo, and A. Amorim. 2005. Mutation rates at Y chromosome specific microsatellites. *Human Mutation* 26: 520–528.

Hammer, M.F., T.M. Karafet, H. Park, K. Omoto, S. Harihara, M. Stoneking, and S. Horai. 2006. Dual origins of the Japanese: Common ground for hunter-gatherer and farmer Y chromosomes. *Journal of Human Genetics* 51: 47–58.

Huang, Y., and H. Li. 2015. Genetic and linguistic evidences suggest a Yeniseian category for Xiongnu. In *Tsinghua Journal of Mongolian History*, vol. 3, ed. Dali Yao, and Yingsheng Liu, 435–456. Beijing: The Commercial Press.

HUGO Pan-Asian SNP Consortium. 2009. Mapping human genetic diversity in Asia. *Science* 326: 1541–1545.

Jobling, M.A., M. Hurles, and C. Tyler-Smith. 2004. *Human evolutionary genetics (origins, peoples and disease)*. New York: Garland Science.

Jobling, M.A., and C. Tyler-Smith. 1995. Father and sons: The Y chromosome and human evolution. *Trends in Genetics* 11: 449–456.

Karafet, T.M., L. Xu, R. Du, W. Wang, S. Feng, R.S. Wells, A.J. Redd, S.L. Zegura, and M.F. Hammer. 2001. Paternal population history of East Asia: Sources, patterns, and microevolutionary processes. *American Journal of Human Genetics* 69 (3): 615–628.

Karafet, T.M., F.L. Mendez, M.B. Meilerman, P.A. Underhill, S.L. Zegura, and M.F. Hammer. 2008. New binary polymorphisms reshape and increase resolution of the human Y chromosomal haplogroup tree. *Genome Research* 18: 830–838.

Kayser, M., S. Brauer, R. Cordaux, A. Casto, O. Lao, L.A. Zhivotovsky, C. Moyse-Faurie, R.B. Rutledge, W. Schiefenhoevel, D. Gil, A.A. Lin, P.A. Underhill, P.J. Oefner, R.J. Trent, and M. Stoneking. 2006. Melanesian and Asian origins of Polynesians: mtDNA and Y chromosome gradients across the Pacific. *Molecular Biology and Evolution* 23: 2234–2244.

Kayser, M., Y. Choi, M. van Oven, S. Mona, S. Brauer, R.J. Trent, D. Suarkia, W. Schiefenhövel, and M. Stoneking. 2008. The impact of the Austronesian expansion: Evidence from mtDNA and Y chromosome diversity in the Admiralty Islands of Melanesia. *Molecular Biology and Evolution* 25 (7): 1362–1374.

Ke, Y., B. Su, X. Song, D. Lu, L. Chen, H. Li, C. Qi, S. Marzuki, R. Deka, P. Underhill, C. Xiao, M. Shriver, J. Lell, D. Wallace, R.S. Wells, M. Seielstad, P. Oefner, D. Zhu, J. Jin, W. Huang, R. Chakraborty, Z. Chen, and L. Jin. 2001. African origin of modern humans in East Asia: A tale of 12,000 Y chromosomes. *Science* 292: 1151–1153.

Kumar, V., A.N. Reddy, J.P. Babu, T.N. Rao, B.T. Langstieh, K. Thangaraj, A.G. Reddy, L. Singh, and B.M. Reddy. 2007. Y-chromosome evidence suggests a common paternal heritage of Austro-Asiatic populations. *BMC Evolutionary Biology* 7: 47.

Li, H., S. Gu, X. Cai, W.C. Speed, A.J. Pakstis, E.I. Golub, J.R. Kidd, and K.K. Kidd. 2008a. Ethnic related selection for an ADH Class I variant within East Asia. *PLoS ONE* 3 (4): e1881.

Li, H., B. Wen, S.J. Chen, B. Su, P. Pramoonjago, Y. Liu, S. Pan, Z. Qin, W. Liu, X. Cheng, N. Yang, X. Li, D. Tran, D. Lu, M.T. Hsu, R. Deka, S. Marzuki, C.C. Tan, and L. Jin. 2008b. Paternal genetic affinity between Western Austronesians and Daic populations. *BMC Evolutionary Biology* 8: 146.

Lu, Y., S.L. Pan, S.M. Qin, Z.D. Qin, C.C. Wang, R.J. Gan, and H. Li. 2013. The Genographic Consortium: Genetic evidence for the multiple origins of Pinghua Chinese. *Journal of Systematics and Evolution* 51 (3): 271–279.

Mirabal, S., M. Regueiro, A.M. Cadenas, L.L. Cavalli-Sforza, P.A. Underhill, D.A. Verbenko, S. A. Limborska, and R.J. Herrera. 2009. Y-chromosome distribution within the geo-linguistic landscape of northwestern Russia. *European Journal of Human Genetics* 17 (10): 1260–1273.

Piazza, A. 1998. Towards a genetic history of China. *Nature* 395: 636–639.

Qin, Z., Y. Yang, L. Kang, S. Yan, K. Cho, X. Cai, Y. Lu, H. Zheng, D. Zhu, D. Fei, S. Li, L. Jin, and H. Li. 2010. A mitochondrial revelation of early human migrations to the Tibetan Plateau before and after the last glacial maximum. *American Journal of Physical Anthropology* 143 (4): 555–569.

Reich, D., R.E. Green, M. Kircher, J. Krause, N. Patterson, E.Y. Durand, B. Viola, A.W. Briggs, U. Stenzel, P.L. Johnson, T. Maricic, J.M. Good, T. Marques-Bonet, C. Alkan, Q. Fu, S. Mallick, H. Li, M. Meyer, E.E. Eichler, M. Stoneking, M. Richards, S. Talamo, M.V. Shunkov, A.P. Derevianko, J.J. Hublin, J. Kelso, M. Slatkin, and S. Pääbo. 2010. Genetic history of an archaic hominin group from Denisova Cave in Siberia. *Nature* 468: 1053–1060.

Rootsi, S., L.A. Zhivotovsky, M. Baldovic, M. Kayser, I.A. Kutuev, R. Khusainova, M.A. Bermisheva, M. Gubina, S.A. Fedorova, A.M. Ilumäe, E.K. Khusnutdinova, M.I. Voevoda, L. P. Osipova, M. Stoneking, A.A. Lin, V. Ferak, J. Parik, T. Kivisild, P.A. Underhill, and R. Villems. 2007. A counter-clockwise northern route of the Y-chromosome haplogroup N from Southeast Asia towards Europe. *European Journal of Human Genetics* 15: 204–211.

Scholes, C., K. Siddle, A. Ducourneau, F. Crivellaro, M. Järve, S. Rootsi, M. Bellatti, K. Tabbada, M. Mormina, M. Reidla, R. Villems, T. Kivisild, M.M. Lahr, and A.B. Migliano. 2011. Genetic diversity and evidence for population admixture in Batak Negritos from Palawan. *American Journal of Physical Anthropology* 146: 62–72.

Sengupta, S., L.A. Zhivotovsky, R. King, S.Q. Mehdi, C.A. Edmonds, C.E. Chow, A.A. Lin, M. Mitra, S.K. Sil, A. Ramesh, M.V. Usha Rani, C.M. Thakur, L.L. Cavalli-Sforza, P.P. Majumder, and P.A. Underhill. 2006. Polarity and temporality of high-resolution y-chromosome distributions in India identify both indigenous and exogenous expansions and reveal minor genetic influence of Central Asian pastoralists. *American Journal of Human Genetics* 78: 202–221.

Shi, Y.F., Z.J. Cui, and J.J. Li. 1989. *Quaternary glacier in eastern China and the climate fluctuation*. Beijing: Science Press.

Shi, H., Y.L. Dong, B. Wen, C.J. Xiao, P.A. Underhill, P.D. Shen, R. Chakraborty, L. Jin, and B. Su. 2005. Y-chromosome evidence of southern origin of the East Asian-specific haplogroup O3-M122. *American Journal of Human Genetics* 77 (3): 408–419.

Shi, H., H. Zhong, Y. Peng, Y.L. Dong, X.B. Qi, F. Zhang, L.F. Liu, S.J. Tan, R.L. Ma, C.J. Xiao, S. Wells, L. Jin, and B. Su. 2008. Y chromosome evidence of earliest modern human settlement in East Asia and multiple origins of Tibetan and Japanese populations. *BMC Biology* 6: 45.

Su, B., J. Xiao, P. Underhill, R. Deka, W. Zhang, J. Akey, W. Huang, D. Shen, D. Lu, J. Luo, J. Chu, J. Tan, P. Shen, R. Davis, L. Cavalli-Sforza, R. Chakraborty, M. Xiong, R. Du, P. Oefner, Z. Chen, and L. Jin. 1999. Y-chromosome evidence for a northward migration of modern human into East Asia during the last ice age. *American Journal of Human Genetics* 65: 1718–1724.

Su, B., L. Jin, P. Underhill, J. Martinson, N. Saha, S.T. McGarvey, M.D. Shriver, J. Chu, P. Oefner, R. Chakraborty, and R. Deka. 2000. Polynesian origins: Insights from the Y chromosome. *Proceedings of the National Academy of Sciences of the United States of America* 97 (15): 8225–8228.

Thangaraj, K., L. Singh, A.G. Reddy, V.R. Rao, S.C. Sehgal, P.A. Underhill, M. Pierson, I.G. Frame, and E. Hagelberg. 2003. Genetic affinities of the Andaman Islanders, a vanishing human population. *Current Biology* 13 (2): 86–93.

Underhill, P.A., P. Shen, A.A. Lin, L. Jin, G. Passarino, W.H. Yang, E. Kauffman, B. Bonné-Tamir, J. Bertranpetit, P. Francalacci, M. Ibrahim, T. Jenkins, J.R. Kidd, S.Q. Mehdi, M.T. Seielstad, R.S. Wells, A. Piazza, R.W. Davis, M.W. Feldman, L.L. Cavalli-Sforza, and P. J. Oefner. 2000. Y chromosome sequence variation and the history of human populations. *Nature Genetics* 26: 358–361.

Wang, C.C., S.E. Farina, and H. Li. 2013a. Neanderthal DNA and modern human origins. *Quaternary International* 295: 126–129.

Wang, C.C., S. Yan, Z.D. Qin, Y. Lu, Q.L. Ding, L.H. Wei, S.L. Li, Y.J. Yang, L. Jin, and H. Li. 2013b. Late Neolithic expansion of ancient Chinese revealed by Y chromosome haplogroup O3a1c-002611. *Journal of Systematics and Evolution* 51 (3): 280–286.

Wen, B., H. Li, D. Lu, X. Song, F. Zhang, Y. He, F. Li, Y. Gao, X. Mao, L. Zhang, J. Qian, J. Tan, J. Jin, W. Huang, R. Deka, B. Su, R. Chakraborty, and L. Jin. 2004a. Genetic evidence supports demic diffusion of Han culture. *Nature* 431: 302–305.

Wen, B., X. Xie, S. Gao, H. Li, H. Shi, X. Song, T. Qian, C. Xiao, J. Jin, B. Su, D. Lu, R. Chakraborty, and L. Jin. 2004b. Analyses of genetic structure of Tibeto-Burman populations reveals sex-biased admixture in southern Tibeto-Burmans. *American Journal of Human Genetics* 74 (5): 856–865.

Xue, Y., Q. Wang, Q. Long, B.L. Ng, H. Swerdlow, J. Burton, C. Skuce, R. Taylor, Z. Abdellah, Y. Zhao, Asan, D.G. MacArthur, M.A. Quail, N.P. Carter, H. Yang, and C. Tyler-Smith. 2009. Human Y chromosome base-substitution mutation rate measured by direct sequencing in a deep-rooting pedigree. *Current Biology* 19 (17): 1453–1457.

Yan, S., C.C. Wang, H. Li, S.L. Li, and L. Jin. 2011. Genographic Consortium: An updated tree of Y-chromosome Haplogroup O and revised phylogenetic positions of mutations P164 and PK4. *European Journal of Human Genetics* 19 (9): 1013–1015.

Zhivotovsky, L.A. 2001. Estimating divergence time with the use of microsatellite genetic distances: Impacts of population growth and gene flow. *Molecular Biology and Evolution* 18: 700–709.

Zhivotovsky, L.A., P.A. Underhill, C. Cinnioğlu, M. Kayser, B. Morar, T. Kivisild, R. Scozzari, F. Cruciani, G. Destro-Bisol, G. Spedini, G.K. Chambers, R.J. Herrera, K.K. Yong, D. Gresham, I. Tournev, M.W. Feldman, and L. Kalaydjieva. 2004. The effective mutation rate at Y chromosome short tandem repeats, with application to human population-divergence time. *American Journal of Human Genetics* 74: 50–61.

Zhong, H., H. Shi, X.B. Qi, C.J. Xiao, L. Jin, R.Z. Ma, and B. Su. 2010. Global distribution of Y-chromosome haplogroup C reveals the prehistoric migration routes of African exodus and early settlement in East Asia. *Journal of Human Genetics* 55 (7): 428–435.

Zhong, H., H. Shi, X.B. Qi, Z.Y. Duan, P.P. Tan, L. Jin, B. Su, and R.Z. Ma. 2011. Extended Y chromosome investigation suggests postglacial migrations of modern humans into East Asia via the northern route. *Molecular Biology and Evolution* 28 (1): 717–727.

Genetic Perspective on Language Replacement in Siberia

Lanhai Wei and Hui Li

1 Introduction

The sharing of language, cultural traditions and/or religion and legends of common ancestors remain as key elements in identifying modern human ethnic groups (Anderson 2006). But as indicated by history, most modern ethnic groups are admixtures of several ancient populations over different historical periods. In recent decades, the Y-chromosome has proven to be a powerful tool in tracing the paternal history of human ethnic groups and genealogical ancestors. The most common scenario is that the distribution of human languages correlates well with Y-chromosome types (indicating male lineages), whereas mtDNA types (associated with maternal descent) don't correlate with languages (Forster and Renfrew 2011). While most ethnic groups from a language branch tend to share the same predominant paternal lineages, there are also exceptions in some cases worldwide.

There are few historical records on the demographic history and languages of the populations living in Siberia. Hence, it is hard to reveal the detailed ethnic history of these populations and the founding process of their languages. A genetic approach will provide a new perspective for such studies. As the language replacement under the elite dominant mode usually took place in very structured

L. Wei (✉) · H. Li (✉)
MOE Key Laboratory of Contemporary Anthropology, School of Life Sciences, Fudan University, Shanghai 200433, People's Republic of China
e-mail: Ryan.lh.Wei@foxmail.com; ryan.lh.wei@gmail.com

H. Li
e-mail: 39232074@qq.com

L. Wei
Institut National des Langues et Civilisations Orientales (INALCO), 63 Rue des Grands Moulins, 75013 Paris, France

D. Xu and H. Li (eds.), *Languages and Genes in Northwestern China and Adjacent Regions*, DOI 10.1007/978-981-10-4169-3_3

populations with a social hierarchy during the historical period (Renfrew 1998), language replacement events or population admixture has left clear genetic mixed signals in the gene pool of present day ethnic groups. We can use genetic signals to assess whether ancient populations interacted. In this study, we have summarized all available Y-SNP haplogroup frequencies for Siberian populations from published research and explored the possible language replacement events in this region. Furthermore, we also briefly discussed the founding process of the Yeniseian language Family, the Altaic language Family (including Turkic, Mongolic, and Tungusic branches), and some other languages.

2 Criteria for Judging Language Replacement

Language replacement, also known as language shift, is a cultural phenomenon in which a human community changes their predominant language to another language, which can be caused by different mechanisms. One of the most common mechanisms is the elite dominant language replacement where a human community gives up their own language and adopts a language with "higher status" in their social hierarchy system (Renfrew 1998). On the other hand, a language replacement can also occur when immigrants reside in a new location that is surrounded by communities speaking another dominant language (hereafter called "integration mode") (Ehret 1988).

In this research, we generally use two policies to demonstrate a language replacement event:

A. For most ethnic groups from a language branch, there is one predominant paternal lineage that had undergone a recent expansion. On the contrary, other ethnic groups from the same language branch have different predominant paternal lineages.
B. For most ethnic groups from a language branch, there are **two or more** predominant paternal lineages that have undergone recent expansions at generally the same historical period. On the contrary, other ethnic groups from the same language branch have different predominant paternal lineages. For this situation, we separate the language replacement into two stages. One of the stages is that language replacement happened before the formation of the common ancestor group of a language branch. In a later period, this language branch spread into a vast geographic region, participating with parallel demic expansions of several predominant paternal lineages. The other stage can be judged by the criterion A.

The comparison of Y-chromosome haplogroup frequencies and the accurate expansion age of paternal lineages in ethnic groups are two key factors in making the judgment of language replacement. In this research, we will also combine achievements from other sub-disciplines of anthropology.

Table 1 Y-chromosome haplogroup frequencies in North Eurasia populations

No.	Ethnic	Language	N	Y* Others	SRY1532.1 BT	M1 DE	M174 D	M130 C	M217 C3*	M48/M77 C3c	M86 C3c1	M407 C3d	FxK	M9 K*	M214 NO*	M175 O	M231 N	LLY22g N1*	P43 N1b	M46 N1c	M45 P*	M242 Q	M207 R*	SRY1532.2 R1a1*	M17 R1a1a	Ref.
1	Saami	U-Saami	23	0	0	8.7	0	0	0	0	0	0	21.7	0	0	0	0	0	0	39.1	0	0	8.7	-	21.7	4
2	Khanty	U-Khanty	28	0	0	0	0	0	0	0	0	0	3.6	0	0	0	0	0	25	64.3	0	0	0	0	7.1	22
3	Khanty	U-Khanty	27	0	0	0	0	0	0	0	0	0	0	0	0	0	0	0	77.8	3.7	0	3.7	0	0	14.8	25
4	Mansi	U-Mansi	25	0	0	0	0	0	0	0	0	0	12	0	0	0	0	0	60	16	0	0	4	0	8	22
5	Nenets	U-Samo.	54	0	0	0	0	0	0	0	0	0	5.6	50	-	0	-	-	-	29.6	0	0	3.7	-	11.1	4
6	Nenets, Forest	U-Samo.	89	1.2	-	-	-	-	-	-	-	-	-	-	0	1.1	0	1.1	44.9	51.7	-	-	-	-	-	30
7	Nenets, Tundra	U-Samo.	59	1.7	-	-	-	-	-	-	-	-	-	-	0	0	0	0	74.6	23.7	-	-	-	-	-	30
8	Selkup	U-Samo.	131	26.7	-	-	-	-	-	-	-	-	-	-	0	0	0	0	6.9	0	-	66.4	-	-	-	30,31
9	Kets	Yeniseian	48	6.2	-	-	-	-	-	-	-	-	-	-	0	0	0	0	0	0	-	93.8	-	-	-	30,31
10	Yakut, Cheriktei	A-Turki.	46	0	0	0	0	2.2	0	0	-	-	0	0	0	0	2.2	-	0	89.1	0	0	0	0	6.5	18
11	Yakut, Byadi	A-Turk.	35	0	0	0	0	0	0	0	0	0	0	0	0	0	0	0	8.6	91.4	0	0	0	0	0	18
12	Yakut, Dyupsya	A-Turk.	28	0	0	0	0	3.6	0	7.1	-	-	0	0	0	0	0	0	0	85.7	0	0	0	0	3.6	18
13	Yakut, cent. okayushie	A-Turk.	49	0	0	0	0	0	2.0	0	0	-	0	0	0	0	0	0	2.0	93.9	0	0	0	0	2.0	19
14	Yakut, cent. akayushie	A-Turk.	47	0	0	0	0	0	2.1	0	0	-	0	0	0	0	0	0	0	93.6	0	0	0	0	4.3	19
15	Yakut, Vilyuy	A-Turk.	56	0	0	0	0	0	0	0	0	0	1.8	0	0	0	0	0	0	98.2	0	0	0	0	0	19
16	Yakut, Northeastern	A-Turk.	32	0	0	0	0	0	3.1	0	3.1	-	0	0	0	0	0	0	0	87.5	0	3.1	0	0	3.1	19
17	Yakut	A-Turk.	46	0	0	0	0	0	0	0	0	0	0	2.2	-	-	4.4	-	-	87	0	0	0	6.52	-	21
18	Yakut	A-Turk.	10	0	0	0	0	0	0	20	-	0	0	0	0	0	0	0	0	80	0	0	0	0	0	14,26
19	Tatar	A-Turk.	126	31.8	-	-	-	1.6	-	-	-	-	-	-	-	-	-	-	4.8	18.3	-	0.8	8.7	34.1	-	24
20	Tatar	A-Turk.	33	0	0	0	0	0	0	0	0	0	33.3	0	-	6.1	0	-	-	-	0	0	0	0	60.6	27
21	Khakassian	A-Turk.	64	48.4	-	-	-	0	1.6	0	0	0	-	-	-	-	-	-	34.4	15.6	-	-	-	-	-	14,26
22	Khakassian	A-Turk.	53	0	0	0	0	5.7	-	-	-	-	3.8	5.7	-	-	-	28.3	-	13.2	7.6	-	7.6	0	28.3	11,12
23	Shor	A-Turk.	51	0	0	0	0	2.0	-	-	-	-	2.0	0	0	0	0	13.7	-	2.0	2.0	-	19.6	0	58.8	11,12
24	Shor	A-Turk.	38	79	-	-	-	0	2.6	0	-	0	-	-	-	-	-	-	15.8	2.6	-	-	-	-	-	14,26
25	Tofalar	A-Turk.	19	0	0	0	0	10.5	-	0	0	-	0	36.8	-	-	-	-	-	47.4	0	0	0	0	5.3	17
26	Tofalar	A-Turk.	32	0	0	0	0	6.3	-	-	-	-	3.1	3.1	-	-	-	34.4	-	25	3.1	-	12.5	0	12.5	11,12
27	Tofalar	A-Turk.	30	30	-	-	-	-	-	-	-	-	-	-	-	-	-	-	43.3	26.7	-	-	-	-	-	26
28	Tuvan-Todjins	A-Turk.	36	0	0	2.8	-	8.3	-	-	-	-	5.6	13.9	-	-	-	2.78	-	11.1	22.2	-	2.8	0	30.6	11,12
29	Tuvan	A-Turk.	51	0	0	0	0	3.9	-	7.8	-	-	5.9	51	-	11.8	-	-	-	2.0	3.9	9.8	2.0	-	2.0	6
30	Tuvan	A-Turk.	51	0	0	0	0	7.8	-	5.9	-	-	5.9	58.8	-	9.8	-	-	-	2.0	3.9	5.9	0	0	0	6
31	Tuvan	A-Turk.	48	0	0	0	0	0	0	4.2	-	0	4.2	14.6	-	2.1	-	-	-	4.2	6.3	62.5	2.1	-	0	6
32	Tuvan	A-Turk.	42	0	0	0	0	9.5	-	7.1	-	-	0	26.2	-	2.4	-	-	-	21.4	16.7	-	2.4	-	14.3	4
33	Tuvan	A-Turk.	40	0	0	2.5	-	10	-	20	-	-	0	27.5	-	-	-	-	-	17.5	15	-	-	-	7.5	17
34	Tuvan	A-Turk.	55	0	0	0	0	0	5.5	0	9.1	-	0	1.8	-	-	-	1.8	27.3	9.1	-	16.4	7.3	-	21.8	19
35	Tuvan	A-Turk.	113	0	0	0.9	-	7.1	-	-	-	-	5.3	8.9	-	-	-	14.2	-	9.7	35.4	-	0.9	0	17.7	11,12
36	Tuvan&Todjins	A-Turk.	134	61.9	-	-	-	0	1.5	6.0	-	1.5	-	-	-	-	-	-	18.7	10.5	-	-	-	-	-	14,26
37	Tuvan-Sojot	A-Turk.	34	0	0	0	0	17.7	-	-	-	-	2.9	26.5	-	-	-	8.8	-	11.8	8.8	-	0	0	23.5	11,12
38	Tuvan-Sojot	A-Turk.	28	35.7	-	-	-	0	0	0	0	53.6	-	-	-	-	-	-	0	10.7	-	-	-	-	-	14,26
39	Kyrgyz	A-Turk.	41	0	7.3	0	0	7.3	-	12.2	-	-	-	2.4	-	-	-	0	0	2.4	4.9	-	-	0	63.4	8
40	Kyrgyz	A-Turk.	13	0	0	0	0	0	7.7	-	-	-	0	30.8	-	-	-	-	-	0	0	0	0	61.5	-	10
41	Kyrgyz	A-Turk.	45	0	0	0	0	8.9	-	-	-	-	0	2.2	-	8.9	4.4	-	-	-	2.2	2.2	2.2	-	68.9	27
42	Kazak	A-Turk.	54	0	-	0	1.9	9.3	-	57.4	-	-	1.9	0	-	11.1	-	-	-	1.9	5.6	-	7.4	-	3.7	4
43	Kazak	A-Turk.	38	0	0	2.6	-	10.5	-	63.2	-	-	0	13.2	-	-	-	0	0	0	7.9	-	-	0	2.6	8
44	Kazak	A-Turk.	30	0	0	0	0	0	40	-	-	-	30	10	-	-	-	-	-	10	3.3	-	6.7	0	0	10
45	Kazak	A-Turk.	41	0	0	0	2.4	58.5	-	-	-	-	9.8	2.4	-	7.3	9.8	-	-	-	0	0	4.9	-	4.9	27
46	Kazakh, Altai	A-Turk.	36	41.7	-	-	-	0	16.7	41.7	-	0	-	-	-	-	-	-	-	-	-	-	-	-	-	14
47	Kazak	A-Turk.	53	0	0	0	1.9	0	75.5	0	0	0	1.9	9.4	-	-	0	0	0	0	-	0	1.9	-	9.4	15,28
48	Uzbek	A-Turk.	28	0	25	3.6	-	14.3	-	0	0	-	-	3.6	-	-	-	0	0	0	21.4	-	-	0	32.1	8
49	Yugur, West	A-Turk.	52	0	0	19.2	-	21.2	-	-	-	-	7.7	48.1	-	-	-	-	-	0	1.9	-	-	0	1.9	23
50	Kalmyk	A-Mong.	99	0	0	1.0	-	24.2	-	37.4	-	-	6.1	13.1	-	-	-	-	-	1.0	11.1	-	6.06	-	0	20
51	Kalmyk	A-Mong.	68	0	0	0	0	70.6	-	-	-	-	0	5.9	-	-	-	2.9	-	0	11.8	-	2.9	0	5.9	11,12
52	Kalmyk	A-Mong.	60	96.7	-	-	-	-	-	-	-	-	-	-	-	-	-	-	3.3	0	-	-	-	-	-	26
53	Kalmyk	A-Mong.	91	37.4	-	-	-	0	5.5	45.1	-	12.1	-	-	-	-	-	-	-	-	-	-	-	-	-	14
54	Kalmyk-Dörwöds	A-Mong.	165	0	0	0	1.2	0	5.5	33.3	-	18.8	2.4	0	0	7.9	0	-	1.2	5.5	0	3.6	17	-	3.6	32
55	Kalmyk-Khoshuuds	A-Mong.	82	0	0	0	0	0	1.2	37.8	-	0	0	0	0	17.1	2.4	-	1.2	36.6	0	1.2	2.4	-	0	32
56	Kalmyk-Torguuds	A-Mong.	150	0	0	0.67	2	0	10.7	46	-	8.7	3.4	0	0	16.7	0	-	1.3	2	0	0.67	3.4	-	4.7	32
57	Khoton	A-Mong.	40	0	0	0	0	0	0	10	-	0	5	0	0	2.5	-	-	-	0	0	0	0	0	82.5	7
58	Mongolian, Uriankhai	A-Mong.	60	0	0	0	1.67	25	-	33.3	-	-	0	5	-	11.7	-	-	-	8.3	8.3	-	-	0	6.7	7
59	Mongolian, Zakhchin	A-Mong.	60	0	0	0	3.3	16.7	-	30	-	-	3.3	5	-	20	-	-	-	3.3	5	-	-	0	13.3	7
60	Mongolian, Khalkh	A-Mong.	48	4.2	-	2.1	-	43.8	-	-	-	-	-	10.4	14.6	25	-	-	-	-	-	-	-	-	-	2

(continued)

Table 1 (continued)

No.	Ethnic	Language	N	Y* Others	SRY1532.1 BT	M1 DE	M174 D	M130 C	M217 C3*	M48M77 C3c	M86 C3c1	M407 C3d	FxK	M9 K*	M214 NO*	M175 O	M231 N	LLY22g N1*	P43 N1b	M46 N1c	M45 P*	M242 Q	M207 R*	SRY1532.2 R1a1*	M17 R1a1a	Ref.
61	Mongolian, Khalkh	A-Mong.	85	0	0	0	3.5	41.2	-	15.3	-	-	4.7	3.5	-	18.8	-	-	-	4.7	4.7	-	-	0	3.5	7
62	Mongolian	A-Mong.	24	0	0	0	4.2	12.5	-	45.8	-	-	8.3	12.5	-	12.5	-	-	-	0	0	0	0	0	4.2	4,5
63	Mongolian	A-Mong.	47	0	0	0	0	57.5	-	-	-	-	2.1	21.3	-	-	-	6.4	-	2.1	4.3	-	4.3	0	2.1	11,12
64	Mongolian	A-Mong.	24	0	0	4.2	-	58.3	-	-	-	-	8.3	12.5	-	12.5	-	-	-	-	0	0	0	0	4.2	1
65	Mongolian	A-Mong.	45	0	4.4	0	-	0	37.8	8.9	-	-	-	4.5	0	31.1	-	0	0	13.3	0	0	0	0	0	3
66	Mongolian	A-Mong.	65	0	6.2	1.5	-	0	33.9	20	-	-	-	1.5	0	12.3	-	0	3.1	7.7	4.6	-	-	0	9.23	3,8
67	Mongolian	A-Mong.	149	0	0	0	2.7	0	34.2	-	18.1	-	4.0	25.5	0.7	-	-	0	6.0	2.0	0	2.7	4.0	-	-	9
68	Mongolian	A-Mong.	147	0	0	0	2.7	0	52.4	-	-	-	4.1	31.3	-	-	-	-	-	2.7	2.7	-	2.0	2.0	-	10
69	Mongolian	A-Mong.	50	0	0	0	4	40	-	-	-	-	0	4	-	38	6	-	-	-	0	2	2	-	4	27
70	Mongolian	A-Mong.	46	26.1	-	-	-	0	39.1	10.9	-	15.2	-	-	-	-	-	-	6.5	2.2	-	-	-	-	-	14,26
71	Mongolian	A-Mong.	22	0	0	0	0	54.6	-	-	-	-	9.1	18.2	-	-	4.6	-	-	-	-	4.6	0	0	9.1	28
72	Mongolian	A-Mong.	12	0	0	0	0	0	25	0	0	0	0	58.3	-	-	8.3	-	-	-	-	0	8.3	-	0	15,28
73	Mongolian	A-Mong.	23	47.8	-	-	-	0	34.8	17.4	-	0	-	-	-	-	-	-	-	-	-	-	-	-	-	15
74	Buryat	A-Mong.	61	0	6.6	0	0	0	83.6	-	-	-	-	0	-	9.84	-	-	-	-	0	0	-	0	0	16
75	Buryat	A-Mong.	50	4	-	4	-	38	-	-	-	-	-	4	30	20	-	-	-	-	-	-	-	-	-	2
76	Buryat	A-Mong.	13	0	0	0	0	0	0	7.69	-	0	7.7	61.5	-	-	-	-	-	23.1	0	0	0	0	0	17
77	Buryat	A-Mong.	81	0	0	0	0	0	55.6	-	4.9	-	2.5	0	0	2.5	-	0	2.5	28.4	0	0	2.5	1.2	-	9,10
78	Buryat	A-Mong.	238	0	0	0	0	63.9	-	-	-	-	2.5	8.8	-	-	-	1.3	-	18.9	1.7	-	0.8	0	2.1	11,12
79	Buryat	A-Mong.	217	12.9	-	-	-	0	8.3	6.0	-	53.9	-	-	-	-	-	-	0.5	18.4	-	-	-	-	-	14,26
80	Khamnigan	A-Mong.	51	46.6	-	-	-	0	0.5	0	-	52.9	-	-	-	-	-	-	-	-	-	-	-	-	-	14
81	Yugur, East	A-Mong.	45	0	0	2.2	-	4.4	-	-	-	-	17.8	15.6	-	44.5	-	-	-	0	13.3	-	-	0	2.2	23
82	Daur	A-Mong.	39	0	5.1	0	-	0	28.2	2.6	-	-	-	0	2.6	53.9	-	0	0	7.7	0	0	0	0	0	3
83	Tu	A-Mong.	50	0	0	0	8	28	-	-	-	-	4	2	-	40	10	-	-	-	0	2	4	-	2	27
84	Evenk, Manchurian	A-Tung.	41	0	0	0	0	0	9.8	-	34.2	-	0	0	0	36.6	-	2.4	2.4	0	0	9.8	0	4.9	-	9,10
85	Evenk	A-Tung.	26	0	0	0	-	3.9	26.9	26.9	-	-	-	3.8	3.9	34.6	-	0	0	0	0	0	0	0	0	3
86	Evenk, Yenisey	A-Tung.	31	0	0	0	0	0	0	58.1	-	0	0	22.6	-	-	-	-	-	9.7	0	0	0	0	9.7	17
87	Evenk	A-Tung.	95	0	-	-	0	0	13.7	-	54.7	-	7.4	0	0	0	-	0	2.1	16.8	0	4.2	1.1	-	-	9
88	Evenk, Yakut speaking	A-Tung.	33	0	0	0	0	0	0	3.0	12.1	0	0	0	0	0	0	0	6.1	72.7	0	0	0	0	6.06	19
89	Evenk, Western	A-Tung.	40	0	0	0	0	0	0	0	70	0	2.5	0	0	0	0	0	27.5	0	0	0	0	0	0	19
90	Evenk	A-Tung.	95	0	0	0	0	0	68.4	-	-	-	7.4	2.1	-	0	-	-	-	16.8	4.2	-	0	1.1	-	10
91	Evenk	A-Tung.	50	0	0	0	0	40	-	-	-	-	6	0	0	0	0	18	-	16	0	0	6	0	14	11,12
92	Evenk	A-Tung.	41	22	-	-	-	0	2.4	43.9	-	2.4	-	-	-	-	-	-	24.4	4.9	-	-	-	-	-	14,26
93	Evenk	A-Tung.	31	0	-	-	0	12.9	-	-	-	-	0	0	-	74.2	12.9	-	-	-	-	0	0	0	0	28
94	Evenk	A-Tung.	57	66.7	-	-	-	0	14	19.3	-	0	-	-	-	-	-	-	-	-	-	-	-	-	-	15
95	Even	A-Tung.	31	0	-	-	0	0	12.9	-	61.3	-	3.2	0	0	0	-	0	0	12.9	0	3.2	6.5	-	-	9
96	Even	A-Tung.	11	90.9	-	-	-	-	-	-	-	-	-	-	-	-	-	-	0	9.1	-	-	-	-	-	26
97	Even	A-Tung.	63	46	-	-	-	0	1.6	52.4	-	0	-	-	-	-	-	-	-	-	-	-	-	-	-	14
98	Orogen	A-Tung.	23	0	0	0	0	0	91.3	-	-	-	0	0	-	4.4	-	-	-	4.4	0	0	0	0	0	10
99	Orogen	A-Tung.	31	0	0	0	-	0	19.4	41.9	-	-	-	3.2	0	29	-	0	6.5	0	0	0	0	0	0	3
100	Orogen	A-Tung.	22	0	-	-	0	0	22.7	-	68.2	-	0	0	0	4.55	-	0	0	4.6	0	0	0	-	-	9
101	Hezhen	A-Tung.	45	0	0	0	-	6.7	11.1	11.1	-	-	-	0	2.2	51.1	-	0	17.8	0	0	0	0	0	0	3
102	Ulchi/Nanai	A-Tung.	53	0	0	0	0	30.2	-	37.7	-	-	0	18.9	-	-	-	-	-	9.4	3.8	-	-	-	0	17
103	Negidal, Upriver	A-Tung.	10	0	0	0	0	0	0	100	-	0	0	0	0	0	0	0	0	0	0	0	0	0	0	17
104	Udegey	A-Tung.	20	0	0	0	0	0	0	60	-	0	0	25	-	-	-	-	-	0	10	-	-	-	5	17
105	Xibo	A-Tung.	41	0	9.8	2.4	-	0	22	4.9	-	-	-	4.9	0	36.6	-	12.2	0	4.9	2.4	-	-	0	0	3
106	Xibo	A-Tung.	32	0	0	0	0	12.5	-	-	-	-	3.1	9.4	-	56.3	15.6	-	-	-	0	0	0	0	3.13	27
107	Xibo	A-Tung.	61	0	0	0	3.3	6.6	29.5	0	0	0	1.6	0	-	39.3	18	-	-	-	-	0	0	0	1.64	15,28
108	Manchu	A-Tung.	18	0	-	0	0	16.7	-	-	-	-	11.1	22.2	-	50	-	-	-	-	0	0	-	-	0	1
109	Manchu	A-Tung.	48	0	-	2.1	-	20.8	-	-	-	-	-	2.1	2.1	72.9	-	-	-	-	-	-	-	-	-	2
110	Manchu	A-Tung.	35	0	0	2.9	-	0	22.9	2.9	-	-	-	2.9	0	54.3	-	11.4	2.9	0	0	0	0	0	0	3
111	Manchu	A-Tung.	52	0	0	0	0	0	26.9	-	0	-	1.92	0	0	57.7	-	5.8	0	0	0	0	5.8	1.9	-	9,10
112	Manchu	A-Tung.	25	56	-	-	-	0	32	12	-	0	-	-	-	-	-	-	-	-	-	-	-	-	-	15
113	Manchu	A-Tung.	111	77.5	-	-	-	0	17.1	0.9	-	4.5	-	-	-	-	-	-	-	-	-	-	-	-	-	15
114	Nivkhi	Isolated	21	0	4.8	0	0	0	38.1	-	-	-	-	0	-	28.6	-	-	-	-	19.1	-	-	9.5	-	16
115	Nivkh	Isolated	17	0	0	0	0	11.8	-	35.3	-	-	0	17.7	-	-	-	-	-	0	35.3	-	-	-	0	17
116	Yukaghir	Isolated	13	0	0	0	0	0	7.7	7.7	15.4	-	7.7	0	0	0	0	0	0	30.8	0	30.8	0	0	0	19
117	Koryak	C-K	27	0	0	0	0	25.9	-	33.3	-	-	0	0	0	0	0	0	0	22.2	18.5	-	-	-	0	17
118	Koryak	C-K	16	75	-	-	-	-	-	-	-	-	-	-	-	-	-	-	0	25	-	-	-	-	-	26
119	Koryak	C-K	39	61.5	-	-	-	0	38.5	-	-	0	-	-	-	-	-	-	-	-	-	-	-	-	-	14
120	Chukchi	C-K	24	0	0	0	0	0	0	4.17	-	0	0	0	0	0	0	0	0	58.3	33.3	-	-	-	4.2	17
121	Uyghur	A-Turk.	33	0	36.4	0	0	15.2	-	3.03	-	-	-	15.2	-	-	-	0	0	0	9.1	-	-	0	21.2	8
122	Uyghur	A-Turk.	67	0	-	-	4.5	1.5	4.5	-	1.5	-	14.9	0	0	17.9	-	3.0	3.0	0	0	3.0	46.3	-	-	9
123	Uyghur	A-Turk.	68	0	0	0	4.4	1.5	5.9	-	-	-	14.7	10.3	-	13.2	-	-	-	0	4.4	-	23.5	22.1	-	10
124	Uyghur	A-Turk.	49	0	0	0	0	6.1	-	-	-	-	28.6	12.2	-	12.2	-	-	-	4.1	8.2	-	-	0	28.6	23
125	Uyghur	A-Turk.	50	0	0	0	2	4	-	-	-	-	42	18	-	10	2	-	-	-	0	4	2	-	16	27
126	Yugur	A-Turk.	32	0	0	0	43.8	3.1	-	-	-	-	12.5	6.3	-	18.8	6.3	-	-	-	0	0	9.4	-	0	27
127	Uyghur	A-Turk.	48	0	-	-	0	6.25	-	-	-	-	27.1	10.4	-	10.4	4.2	-	-	-	-	2.1	10.4	-	29.2	28
128	Uyghur	A-Turk.	71	2.8	-	-	1.4	7.0	-	-	-	-	18.3	2.8	-	12.7	4.2	-	-	-	-	8.5	7.0	-	35.2	28
129	Uyghur	A-Turk.	18	5.6	-	-	5.6	0	-	-	-	-	22.2	0	-	27.8	5.6	-	-	-	-	5.6	5.6	-	22.2	28
130	Uyghur	A-Turk.	50	0	-	-	8	8	-	-	-	-	16	4	-	14	6	-	-	-	-	6	14	-	24	28
131	Uyghur	A-Turk.	187	93.1	-	-	-	1	4.3	0.5	-	1.1	-	-	-	-	-	-	-	-	-	-	-	-	-	15

Abbreviation for language classification U-Saami for Saami group of Uralic; *U-Khanty* for Khanty group of Uralic; *U-Mansi* for Mansi group of Uralic; *U-Samo* for Samoyed group of Uralic; *A-Turk* for Turkic group of Altaic; *A-Mong* for Mongolic group of Altaic; *A-Tung* for Tungusic group of Altaic; *C-K* for Chukchi-Kamchatkan

3 Summary of Paternal Genetic Data

To obtain a comprehensive picture of the paternal gene pool of Siberian populations, Y-chromosome haplogroup frequencies of 131 populations living in Siberia or nearby regions were collected from the literature (Chen et al. 2011; Derenko et al. 2006a; b, 2007; Hammer et al. 2006; Hong et al. 2006; Karafet et al. 2001, 2002; Katoh et al. 2005; Khar'kov et al. 2008; Lell et al. 2002; Malyarchuk et al. 2010, 2013; Mirabal et al. 2009; Nasidze et al. 2005; Pakendorf et al. 2006; Pimenoff et al. 2008; Puzyrev et al. 2003; Rootsi et al. 2007; Shi et al. 2008; Shou et al. 2010; Su et al. 1999; Tajima et al. 2004; Tambets et al. 2004; Wells et al. 2001; Xue et al. 2006; Zerjal et al. 2002; Zhong et al. 2010, 2011; Zhou et al. 2008) (Table 1). Since the tested Y-SNP markers varied in different research, we aligned the frequencies of Y-chromosome haplogroups according to the phylogenetic tree on http://www.isogg.org. Based on the comparison of Y-chromosome haplogroup frequencies and the expansion age of each paternal lineage, we will discuss possible language replacement events in Siberia in the following sections.

4 Possible Yeniseian Origin of Selkup

The Selkup language belongs to the Samoyed branch of the Uralic language Family (Lewis et al. 2015). The Selkups live by the Taz River and between the middle reaches of the Ob and the Yenisey in Siberia (Kolga et al. 2013). According to previous research, Y-chromosome lineages N1b-P43 and N1c-M178 are two predominant paternal lineages of Uralic-speaking populations (Rootsi et al. 2007), as shown in Table 1. The highest frequencies of haplogroup N1b-P43 were observed in Samoyed populations, like Ngansan (91.1%) and Nenets (74.6%). This haplogroup is also the dominant paternal lineage of Khanty and Mansi populations. On the contrary, Selkups have minor percent of N1b-P43 (6.9%), while haplogroup Q-M242 (66.4%) is the most frequent paternal lineage in this population. Moreover, haplogroup Q is the predominant lineage of the Kets (93.8%), the only living group of the Yeniseian language family. Haplogroup Q-M242 and haplogroup N1b/N1c split around 50,000 years ago. These two haplogroups represent different demographic histories in different regions of the Eurasian continent.

Genetic data shows that the Q-M242 clade in Selkups is one branch of Q1a3a3-L330 found in the Kets population. As seen in Fig. 1, the total age of haplogroup Q1a3a3-B287 is about 5000 years, while the Selkup sample split from the Kets sample at a relatively late age (about 2700 years ago). Given the fact that the Yeniseian language once spread widely along the Yenisei River and the Selkup's range is close to the Yenisai River, it's highly likely that the Selkup population originated from a Yeniseian-speaking group. After their migration into the settlement region of Samoyed populations, they changed their language at an unknown historical period.

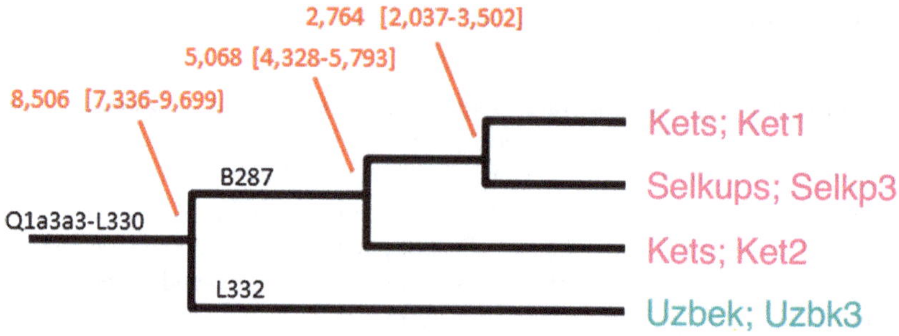

Fig. 1 Phylogenetic tree of paternal lineage Q1a3a3-L330 in Kets and Selkups, based on full Y-chromosome sequences. Number in red indicates the splitting time of downstream branches. Modified from figure S3 of Karmin et al. (2015)

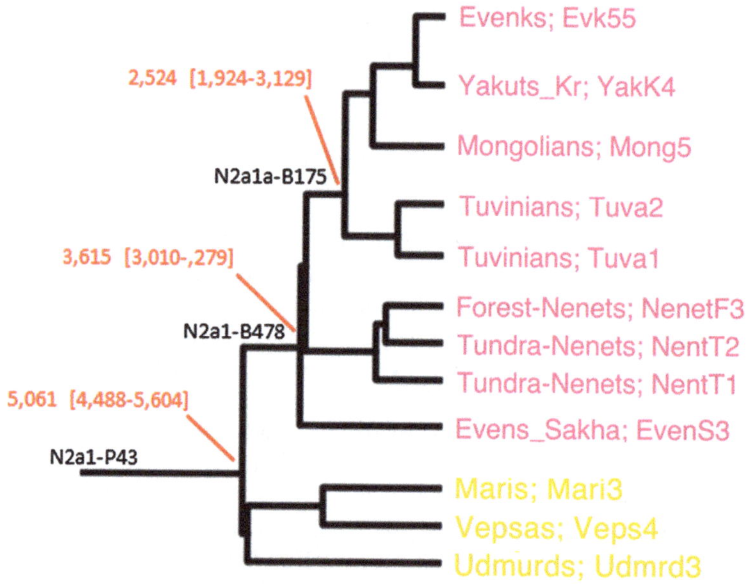

Fig. 2 Phylogenetic tree of N1b-P43 in Samoyed, Tuvan, and other populations, based on full Y-chromosome sequences. Numbers in red indicate the splitting time of downstream branches. Modified from figure S3 of Karmin et al. (2015)

5 Khakassian and Shors

There are four predominant paternal lineages in these two populations, including N1b-P43, N1c-M178, Q-M242, and R1a1a-M17. According to previous research, N1c-M178 and Q-M242 may have lived in south Siberia since the Paleolithic age (Dulik et al. 2012; Rootsi et al. 2007). In addition, ancient DNA shows that haplogroup R1a1a-M17 has been the predominant lineage in the Altai Mountain region since the Andronovo Culture period (Keyser et al. 2009). Nowadays, there is no Samoyed-speaking population in the Minusinsk Basin and Sayan mountain region. But some ethnology books record that there were some Samoyed tribes classified as Southern Samoyed in the Minusinsk Basin and Tuva until the 17 century (Hajdú 1968; Potapov 1969). They became extinct during later periods. From a genetic perspective, N1b-P43 samples in Samoyed and Tuvan populations belong to a specific sub-clade named N2a1-B478. The expansion time of N2a1-B478 is only about 3600 years ago, as shown in Fig. 2. Hence, we propose that the southern part of Samoyed populations may have changed their language to a Turkic language at various historical periods, bringing haplogroup N2a1-B478 into Tuvan, Khakassian, and Shors populations.

6 The Tuvans and Tofalars

The Tofalars live in the northern region of the East Sayan Mountains. They are assumed to be close relatives of Tuvans. Also, some research lists Todjins and Sojots as separate ethnic groups distinct from the Tuvans. But usually these two groups are considered as clans of the Tuvans (Vainshtein 1980). According to the 16 sets of data in Table 1, the frequencies of the Y-SNP haplogroup varied a lot in Tuvans samples from different research. Haplogroups N1b-P43, Q-M242, R1a1a-M17, and N1c-M46 can be considered as predominant paternal lineages in Tuvan populations. Additionally, lineage C3-M217 (or C-M130) is quite frequent in Tuvan populations. The Tofalar paternal gene pool is similar to that of the Tuvans. On the contrary, Tuvan-Sojots was found to have a high frequency of C3d-M407 in reference 17.

The high diversities of paternal lineages among the Tuvans and Tofalars are consistent with the complex demographic history of South Siberia, especially the Sayan Mountain and Altaic Mountain region. Previous research showed that Paleolithic populations in South Siberia may be ancestors of most modern ethnic groups in North Eurasia and of Native Americans (Raghavan et al. 2014). Many ancient populations once lived in this region, including populations of the Afanasievo Culture, Andronovo Culture, Chermurchek Culture, and a series of succeeding cultures. In the recent historical period, various populations have lived in this region, including Yeniseian, Samoyed, Turkic, and Mongolic populations. All these populations should have left genetic signals among the Tuvans, Tofalars, and their relatives. Therefore, language replacement may have occurred many times during the historical period in this region.

As discussed in the section on the Khakassian and Shors, some of ancient southern Samoyed populations may have changed their language to the Tuvan language and became part of Tuvan populations. More Y-chromosome sequencing data are needed to reveal a clearer scenario of demographic and linguistic transition in this region since ancient times. Since the C3d-M407 haplotype of the Tuvan-Sojots belongs to the Buryats special lineage and the genetic diversity of

C3d-M407 in Tuvan-Sojots is extremely low, we can assume that a Mongolic-speaking population group (possible Buryats) may have changed their language to a Turkic language when they moved westward into the Sayan Mountain region and finally became a part of Tuvan populations.

7 Kyrgyz and Kazak

The predominant paternal lineage of the Kyrgyz is R1a1a-M17, as seen in Table 1. Karmin et al. 2015 showed that R1a1a-M17 samples in Kyrgyz are classified into two sub-clades (Karmin et al. 2015). One is R1a2a2-B116, a brother branch of R1a2a2-B115 in Altain populations. The other lineage is R1a2c'd-Z2125 which is distributed widely in populations from Central Asia, South Asia and the Middle East. Additional unpublished data from our lab shows that the N1b-P43 and C3*-Star clusters are also important Kyrgyz lineages. We propose that R1a2a2-B116 and N1b-P43 represent the connection of Kyrgyz with populations in South Siberia. On the contrary, R1a2c'd-Z2125 and C3*-Star cluster represent admixture after their migration into the region where they currently reside. More importantly, the Fuyu Kyrgyz language, found in Fuyun County in Heilongjiang province of China, is close to the Khakas language of South Siberia. Since historical records show that present-day Kyrgyz in Kirgizstan originated from the South Siberian region, we propose that the original language of Kyrgyz in Kirgizstan was close to some Turkic languages in South Siberia (perhaps from the "Northern cluster" of the Turkic language group). After their migration to the region where they currently reside, their language changed and became close to Kazak, which belongs to the "Western cluster" of the Turkic language group.

For Kazak populations, a high frequency of haplogroup C3*-M217 can be observed in nearly all research, as seen in Table 1. Further studies showed that most C3*-M217 samples in Kazaks belong to the C3-Star cluster (Abilev et al. 2012). The distribution of this lineage in Eurasia had been proposed to be associated with activities of Chengisz Khan or his close relatives (Zerjal et al. 2002). As summarized in unpublished research at our lab, C3-Star cluster samples in Kazaks are related to Mongolic tribes in the Eastern Chagatai Khanate (A.D. 1348–1514). During the founding process of the Kazak Khanate, a number of Mongol tribes in Eastern Chagatai Khanate moved to the west and joined the Kazak Khanate alliance where a Turkic language (the Kazak language) is the official one. More recently, they have become important parts of modern Kazak populations. Nowadays, the tribal structure is still very strong among Kazaks. So, we propose that the high frequency of the C3-Star cluster was brought in a language replacement event by Mongolic-speaking tribes during the founding process of the modern Kazak ethnicity. Admixture of language elements may also have occurred during the integration of different ethnic groups. From a genetic perspective, it's unreasonable to trace the common words from the Turkic language group and the Mongolic language group in the modern Kazak language.

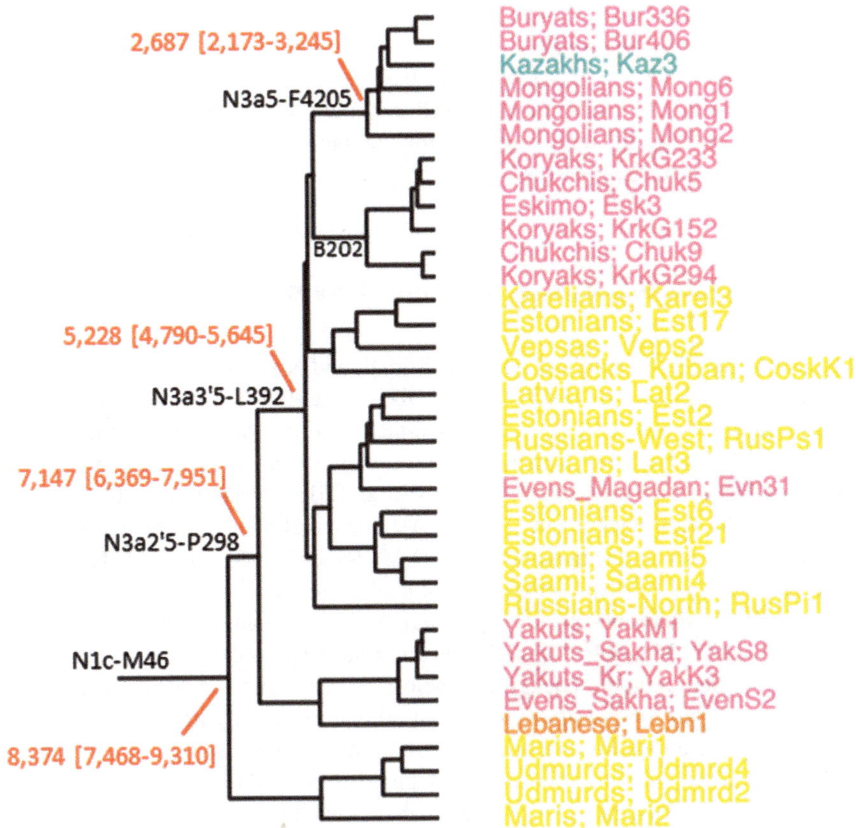

Fig. 3 Phylogenetic tree of paternal lineage N1c-M46 in North Eurasian populations, based on full Y-chromosome sequences. Numbers in red indicate the splitting time of downstream branches. Modified from figure S3 of Karmin et al. (2015)

8 Yakuts

As seen in Table 1, N1c-M46 is the predominant paternal lineage in Yakut populations. Samples of N1c-M46 among Yakuts belong to a special sub-clade named N3a2'5-P298 (Karmin et al. 2015). This sub-clade split from its brother branch N3a1-B211 about 7000 years ago, as shown in Fig. 3. On the contrary, most N1c-M46 samples in Turkic and Mongolic populations belong to another lineage (N3a1-B211). According to archaeological studies, remains of an ancient seminomadic population from the Lake Baikal region, identified as the Turkic-speaking Kurykan people, exhibit close affinities to Yakut culture (Konstantinov 1975; Okladnikov 1970). Hence, it's generally accepted that Yakut populations are descendants of Turkic-speaking populations in the south of their present-day living region. However, N1c-M46 only comprises a minor part or zero present of paternal lineages in other Turkic populations. As proposed by linguists, diffusion of the Turkic language was largely a result of an "elite dominant mode" during the Turkic Khanate period (A.D. 552–744). Although the paternal lineages of the ruling family of the Turkic Khanate (Ashina clan) is still unknown, we propose that ancestors of Yakut may have changed their language from an unknown one to a Turkic language at an unknown historical period.

9 Mongolian, Kalmyk, Buryat and Khamnigan

As seen in Table 1, Mongolian, Kalmyk, Buryat, and Khamnigan populations have three predominant paternal lineages: C3*-M217, C3c-M48, and C3d-M407. Deep research indicates that most C3*-M217 samples in Mongolic-speaking populations belong to C3-Star cluster which was considered to be the paternal lineage of Chengis Khan or his relatives (Malyarchuk et al. 2013; Zerjal et al. 2002). Hence, we propose that this clade is the core paternal lineage of Mongolic populations. On the other hand, other lineages including D-M174, O-M175, N1b-P43, N1c-M46, Q-M242 and R-M207 also comprise considerable frequencies in the paternal gene pools of these Mongolic-speaking populations. Since many ancient populations once lived on the Mongolian Plateau and Eurasian steppe, these haplogroups may represent the demographic background before the expansion of Mongolian. Also, we cannot rule out the possibility of recent admixture during the historical period from other populations into Mongolic-speaking populations.

For Buryat populations, the high frequency of N1c-M46 can be observed in samples from all research. According to their own history, the original Buryat alliance consisted of the Khori-Tumed tribe, the Bargu tribe and some other hunter-gatherer clans (Abide 1982). The ancient "Bargu" tribe was considered to be a descendant of the Bayarqu (or Bayegu/Baiyrku), a Turkic-speaking tribe in the Turkic Khanate (Tsydendambaev 1972). On the other hand, "Tumed" is possibly an ancient Monglic word. So, we propose that a Turkic-speaking population (a.k. Bayarqu->Bargu) changed their language and finally became an important part of modern Buryat populations.

The history of the Khamnigan (or Hamnigan), a Mongolic-speaking population living near Nerchinsk, remains unambiguous. Ethnologists believe that the Khamnigans originated from the Tungusic speaking Evenks tribe and underwent Mongolization in the early 16th century (Shubin 1973). But according to genetic data, Khamnigans have a high frequency of C3d-M407 (52.9%) and they do not have haplogroup C3c-M48 which is the predominant lineage of Tungusic speaking populations. We can also predict that the Khamnigan should have a high frequency of N1c-M46 (33.3%), given the Y-chromosome haplotype of this population (Malyarchuk et al. 2013). The two predominant lineages in Khamnigan, C3d-M407 and N1c-M46, make them very close to the Buryat population. Hence, we propose that the Khamnigan were probably originally a Mongolic-speaking population (close to ancestor of Buryats). It may be unreasonable to argue the Tungusic origin of this population. But on the other hand, we cannot rule out the possibility that they changed to a Tungusic language at an unknown historical period and underwent a re-Mongolization process in the early 16th century.

10 Evenks and Evens

Evenks and Evens were indigenous populations in Siberia before the expansion of Yakuts, living in a vast region ranging from Kamchatka Peninsula in the East to Tunguska River region in the West (Naumov 2006). All available data indicate that haplogroup C3c-M48 is the predominant paternal lineage of Evenks and Evens, as well as other Tungusic-speaking populations. But Yakut-speaking Evenks from Pakendorf et al. 2006 have high frequency of N1c-M46 (72.7%) and low frequency of C3c-M48 (12.1%) (Pakendorf et al. 2006). This population traces their ancestors to the Yakuts, but their claimed ethnicity is currently Evenk. This an interesting case of ethnic identification caused by immigration and intermarriage.

11 Koryak and Chukchi

Two major lineages, N1c-M46 and Q-M242, were observed in the Chukchi population. Besides these two lineages, C3*-M217 also comprise a considerable frequncy in the Koryak paternal gene pool. Deep sequencing indicated that these C3*-M217 samples in Koryaks belong to C3c2-B90, a rare lineage found in the Evenks and Yakuts. This rare lineage may represent the remains of an ancient population in Northeast Asia.

12 Manchu and Other Tungusic-Speaking Populations

Similar to the situation of the Evenks and Evens in Siberia, C3c-M48 is also the predominant paternal lineage in Tungusic-speaking populations living in the Amur River region (Heilongjiang River in Chinese), including the Oroqen, Hezhen, Nanai, Negidal, Udegey etc. The only exception is Manchu (see Table 1). In Manchu, the frequency of C3c-M48 is low and there is high frequency of haplogroup O-M175. This is consistent with the intense admixture between the Manchu and Han Chinese ethnicities. An interesting fact was found when we started to study the paternal lineage of Aisin Gioro, the imperial house of the Qing dynasty which was founded by the Manchu ethnicity. The paternal lineage of Aisin Gioro is confirmed to be C3b2b1*-M401 (xF5483) rather than C3c-M48(Yan et al. 2015). Further sequencing showed that this lineage is the brother branch of C3-Star cluster which was considered to be the clade of Chengis Khan or his close relatives (unpublished date from our lab). This finding is unexpected, but may be consistent with the legend of the Aisin Gioro clan regarding their origin. As argued by a textual research(Yao and Sun 2012), the origin location of the Aisin Gioro clan is not Baekdu Mountain (Changbai Mountain in Chinese) as they claimed, but the border region of the middle reaches of the Amur River near Heihe City in Heilongjiang Province, China. This city, which used to be called Aihui City, was surrounded by Daur populations from the 14th century to the 17th century. Regarding the genetic data on this connection, we do find higher frequency of potential C3b2b1*-M401 (xF5483) samples in Daur populations based on Y-STR haplotypes from Lihong Zheng et al. (2009). Y-SNP testing of Daur population samples is needed to confirm this STR prediction. Beside the legend mentioned above, there are no official history records on the early history of the Aisin Gioro clan. Hence, according to genetic data, we propose that the Aisin Gioro clan probably changed their language from a Daur-like language to a Tungusic language during the long-distance migration from the border region of the middle reaches of the Amur River to Hetuela City in Liaoning Province, China.

13 Discussion

According to the latest achievements of genetic studies, there are s founding paternal lineages for Uralic populations: N2a1-L1419, N2a1a-B169, N3a1-B211, N3a3a-L550, N3a3b-VL39, and N3a4-Z1936. More studies on the expansion times of these lineages and sampling from a vast region are needed to explore the detailed ethnic history of Uralic populations and the founding process of this language family. In North Eurasian populations, there are some other brother branches of these lineages. These lineages represent the demographic background of North Eurasia. Most of them have become important parts of other modern ethnic groups in Siberia. So, they are keys to understanding the history of Turkic and Mongolic-speaking populations and their languages.

Until now, the available genetic data is not detailed enough to determine the founding paternal lineages of Turkic language group populations. Various predominant lineages were observed in different Turkic-speaking populations, such as Q-M25 in Turkmen, C3*-Star cluster in Kazaks, R1a1a–M17 in Kyrgyz and populations in Altai Mountain Region, N1b-P43 and Q-L53 in Tuvan/Tofalar and N1c-M46 in Yakuts. The genetic pattern we have now observed is extremely consistent with the proposed "elite dominant mode" for expansion of Turkic languages. Ancient DNA may help to understand the early history of Turkic-speaking populations and their languages.

For Mongolic-speaking populations, current genetic data shows that there were three founding paternal lineages, including C3*-F1918 (previously known as Star Cluter), C3c-M48, and C3d-M407. Haplogroup C3-F1756, characterized by a deletion on DYS448, is also distributed widely in Mongolic-speaking populations, even though its frequency is low. According to the available data, these four lineages originated from different regions before they integrated and became a common ancestor group of all present-day Mongolic-speaking populations. More work on these four lineages and ancient DNA tests are needed to understand the detailed history of Mongolic-speaking populations and their languages.

There is little Y-chromosome sequencing data for Koryak and Chukchi populations. These two populations are generally admixtures of ancient populations with predominant lineage Q-M242 and ancient populations with predominant lineage N1c-M46. The N1c-M46 clade in Koryak, Chukchi, and Eskimo populations split from its brother clade at about 4900 years ago and started its expansion about 2700 years ago, as shown in Fig. 3.

In conclusion, the current available genetic evidence from Siberian populations outlines a general scenario of dispersal and expansion patterns of various paternal lineages throughout Siberia. Populations from the same language group tend to have their own predominant paternal lineages. In this research, based on the comparison of Y-chromosome haplogroup frequencies and dating of each sub-clade among different populations, we proposed a series of language replacement events during the founding of Siberian populations and their language family and/or group. However, sequencing more samples from ethnic groups and testing ancient DNA are needed to form a solid conclusion about the complex demographic history of Siberian populations and their languages.

References

Abide, B. 1982. *Brief history of Buryat Mongolian*. Hulunbuir: Inner Mongolia Cultural Publishing House.

Abilev, S., B. Malyarchuk, M. Derenko, M. Wozniak, T. Grzybowski, and I. Zakharov. 2012. The Y-chromosome C3* star-cluster attributed to Genghis Khan's descendants is present at high frequency in the Kerey clan from Kazakhstan. *Human Biology* 84: 79–89. doi:10.3378/027.084.0106.

Anderson, B. 2006. *Imagined communities: Reflections on the origin and spread of nationalism*, Revised edition. London: Verso.

Chen, Z., Y. Zhang, A. Fan, Y. Zhang, Y. Wu, Q. Zhao, Y. Zhou, C. Zhou, M. Bawudong, X. Mao, Y. Ma, L. Yang, Y. Ding, X. Wang, and S. Rao. 2011. Brief communication: Y-chromosome haplogroup analysis indicates that Chinese Tuvans share distinctive affinity with Siberian Tuvans. *American Journal of Physical Anthropology* 144: 492–497. doi:10.1002/ajpa.21453.

Derenko, M., B. Malyarchuk, G.A. Denisova, M. Wozniak, I. Dambueva, C. Dorzhu, F. Luzina, D. Miscicka-Sliwka, and I. Zakharov. 2006a. Contrasting patterns of Y-chromosome variation in South Siberian populations from Baikal and Altai-Sayan regions. *Human Genetics* 118: 591–604. doi:10.1007/s00439-005-0076-y.

Derenko, M.V., B.A. Malyarchuk, M. Wozniak, I.K. Dambuveva, C.M. Dorzhu, F.A. Luzina, H.K. Lee, D. Miscicka-Sliwka, and I.A. Zakharov. 2006b. The diversity of Y-chromosome lineages in indigenous population of South Siberia. *Doklady Biological Sciences* 411: 466–470.

Derenko, M., B. Malyarchuk, G. Denisova, M. Wozniak, T. Grzybowski, I. Dambueva, and I. Zakharov. 2007. Y-chromosome haplogroup N dispersals from south Siberia to Europe. *Journal of Human Genetics* 52: 763–770. doi:10.1007/s10038-007-0179-5.

Dulik, M.C., S.I. Zhadanov, L.P. Osipova, A. Askapuli, L. Gau, O. Gokcumen, S. Rubinstein, and T.G. Schurr. 2012. Mitochondrial DNA and Y chromosome variation provides evidence for a recent common ancestry between Native Americans and Indigenous Altaians. *American Journal of Human Genetics* 90: 229–246. doi:10.1016/j.ajhg.2011.12.014.

Ehret, C. 1988. Language change and the material correlates of language and ethnic shift. *Antiquity* 62: 564–574. doi:10.1017/S0003598X00074731.

Forster, P., and C. Renfrew. 2011. Evolution. Mother tongue and Y chromosomes. *Science* 333: 1390–1391. doi:10.1126/science.1205331.

Hajdú, P. 1968. *The Samoyed peoples and languages*. Bloomington: Indiana University.

Hammer, M.F., T.M. Karafet, H. Park, K. Omoto, S. Harihara, M. Stoneking, and S. Horai. 2006. Dual origins of the Japanese: Common ground for hunter-gatherer and farmer Y chromosomes. *Journal of Human Genetics* 51: 47–58. doi:10.1007/s10038-005-0322-0.

Hong, S., H. Jin, K.D. Kwak, W. Kim. 2006. Y-chromosome haplogroup O3-M122 variation in East Asia and its implications for the peopling of Korea. *Korean Journal of Genetics* 28: 1–8.

Karafet, T., L. Xu, R. Du, W. Wang, S. Feng, R.S. Wells, A.J. Redd, S.L. Zegura, and M.F. Hammer. 2001. Paternal population history of East Asia: Sources, patterns, and microevolutionary processes. *American Journal of Human Genetics* 69: 615–628. doi:10.1086/323299.

Karafet, T.M., L.P. Osipova, M.A. Gubina, O.L. Posukh, S.L. Zegura, and M.F. Hammer. 2002. High levels of Y-chromosome differentiation among native Siberian populations and the genetic signature of a boreal hunter-gatherer way of life. *Human Biology* 74: 761–789.

Karmin, M., L. Saag, M. Vicente, M.A. Wilson Sayres, M. Jarve, U.G. Talas, S. Rootsi, A.M. Ilumae, R. Magi, M. Mitt, L. Pagani, T. Puurand, Z. Faltyskova, F. Clemente, A. Cardona, E. Metspalu, H. Sahakyan, B. Yunusbayev, G. Hudjashov, M. DeGiorgio, E.L. Loogvali, C. Eichstaedt, M. Eelmets, G. Chaubey, K. Tambets, S. Litvinov, M. Mormina, Y. Xue, Q. Ayub, G. Zoraqi, T.S. Korneliussen, F. Akhatova, J. Lachance, S. Tishkoff, K. Momynaliev, F.X. Ricaut, P. Kusuma, H. Razafindrazaka, D. Pierron, M.P. Cox, G.N. Sultana, R. Willerslev, C. Muller, M. Westaway, D. Lambert, V. Skaro, L. Kovacevic, S. Turdikulova, D. Dalimova, R. Khusainova, N. Trofimova, V. Akhmetova, I. Khidiyatova, D.V. Lichman, J. Isakova, E. Pocheshkhova, Z. Sabitov, N.A. Barashkov, P. Nymadawa, E. Mihailov, J.W. Seng, I. Evseeva, A.B. Migliano, S. Abdullah, G. Andriadze, D. Primorac, L. Atramentova, O. Utevska, L. Yepiskoposyan, D. Marjanovic, A. Kushniarevich, D.M. Behar, C. Gilissen, L. Vissers, J.A. Veltman, E. Balanovska, M. Derenko, B. Malyarchuk, A. Metspalu, S. Fedorova, A. Eriksson, A. Manica, F.L. Mendez, T.M. Karafet, K.R. Veeramah, N. Bradman, M.F. Hammer, L.P. Osipova, O. Balanovsky, E.K. Khusnutdinova, K. Johnsen, M. Remm, M.G. Thomas, C. Tyler-Smith, P.A. Underhill, E. Willerslev, R. Nielsen, M. Metspalu, R. Villems, and T. Kivisild. 2015. A recent bottleneck of Y chromosome diversity coincides with a global change in culture. *Genome Research* 25: 459–466. doi:10.1101/gr.186684.114.

Katoh, T., B. Munkhbat, K. Tounai, S. Mano, H. Ando, G. Oyungerel, G.T. Chae, H. Han, G. J. Jia, K. Tokunaga, N. Munkhtuvshin, G. Tamiya, and H. Inoko. 2005. Genetic features of Mongolian ethnic groups revealed by Y-chromosomal analysis. *Gene* 346: 63–70. doi:10.1016/j.gene.2004.10.023.

Keyser, C., C. Bouakaze, E. Crubezy, V.G. Nikolaev, D. Montagnon, T. Reis, and B. Ludes. 2009. Ancient DNA provides new insights into the history of south Siberian Kurgan people. *Human Genetics* 126: 395–410. doi:10.1007/s00439-009-0683-0.

Khar'kov, V.N., V.A. Stepanov, O.F. Medvedev, M.G. Spiridonova, N.R. Maksimova, A.N. Nogovitsyna, and V.P. Puzyrev. 2008. The origin of Yakuts: Analysis of Y-chromosome haplotypes. *Molecular Biology (Mosk)* 42: 226–237.

Kolga, M., I. Tõnurist, L. Vaba, J. Viikberg. 2013. *The red book of the peoples of the Russian Empire*. Thomas Niimann.

Konstantinov, I.V. 1975. *The origins of the Yakut people and their culture: Yakutia and her neighbors in antiquity*. Yakutsk: Yakutskiy filial SO AN SSSR. [in Russian].

Lell, J.T., R.I. Sukernik, Y.B. Starikovskaya, B. Su, L. Jin, T.G. Schurr, P.A. Underhill, and D.C. Wallace. 2002. The dual origin and Siberian affinities of Native American Y chromosomes. *American Journal of Human Genetics* 70: 192–206. doi:10.1086/338457.

Lewis, M.P., G.F. Simons, C.D. Fennig. 2015. *Ethnologue: Languages of the world*. Dallas, Texas: SIL International.

Malyarchuk, B., M. Derenko, G. Denisova, M. Wozniak, T. Grzybowski, I. Dambueva, and I. Zakharov. 2010. Phylogeography of the Y-chromosome haplogroup C in northern Eurasia. *Annals of Human Genetics* 74: 539–546. doi:10.1111/j.1469-1809.2010.00601.x.

Malyarchuk, B., M. Derenko, G. Denisova, S. Khoyt, M. Wozniak, T. Grzybowski, and I. Zakharov. 2013. Y-chromosome diversity in the Kalmyks at the ethnical and tribal levels. *Journal of Human Genetics* 58: 804–811. doi:10.1038/jhg.2013.108.

Mirabal, S., M. Regueiro, A.M. Cadenas, L.L. Cavalli-Sforza, P.A. Underhill, D.A. Verbenko, S. A. Limborska, and R.J. Herrera. 2009. Y-chromosome distribution within the geo-linguistic landscape of northwestern Russia. *European Journal of Human Genetics* 17: 1260–1273. doi:10.1038/ejhg.2009.6.

Nasidze, I., D. Quinque, I. Dupanloup, R. Cordaux, L. Kokshunova, and M. Stoneking. 2005. Genetic evidence for the Mongolian ancestry of Kalmyks. *American Journal of Physical Anthropology* 128: 846–854. doi:10.1002/ajpa.20159.

Naumov, I.V. 2006. *The history of Siberia*. London: Routledge.

Okladnikov, A.P. 1970. *Yakutia: Before its incorporation into the Russian state*. Montreal: McGill-Queen's University Press.

Pakendorf, B., I.N. Novgorodov, V.L. Osakovskij, A.P. Danilova, A.P. Protod'jakonov, and M. Stoneking. 2006. Investigating the effects of prehistoric migrations in Siberia: Genetic variation and the origins of Yakuts. *Human Genetics* 120: 334–353. doi:10.1007/s00439-006-0213-2.

Pimenoff, V.N., D. Comas, J.U. Palo, G. Vershubsky, A. Kozlov, and A. Sajantila. 2008. Northwest Siberian Khanty and Mansi in the junction of West and East Eurasian gene pools as revealed by uniparental markers. *European Journal of Human Genetics* 16: 1254–1264. doi:10.1038/ejhg.2008.101.

Potapov, L.P. 1969. *Ocherki narodnogo byta tuvintsev (Essays on the traditional life of Tuvinians)*. Moscow: Nauka.

Puzyrev, V.P., V.A. Stepanov, M.V. Golubenko, K.V. Puzyrev, N.R. Maksimova, V.N. Khar'kov, M.G. Spiridonova, and A.N. Nogovitsyna. 2003. MtDNA and Y-chromosome lineages in the Yakut population. *Genetika* 39: 975–981.

Raghavan, M., P. Skoglund, K.E. Graf, M. Metspalu, A. Albrechtsen, I. Moltke, S. Rasmussen, T. W. Stafford Jr., L. Orlando, E. Metspalu, M. Karmin, K. Tambets, S. Rootsi, R. Magi, P.F. Campos, E. Balanovska, O. Balanovsky, E. Khusnutdinova, S. Litvinov, L.P. Osipova, S.A. Fedorova, M.I. Voevoda, M. DeGiorgio, T. Sicheritz-Ponten, S. Brunak, S. Demeshchenko, T. Kivisild, R. Villems, R. Nielsen, M. Jakobsson, and E. Willerslev. 2014. Upper Palaeolithic Siberian genome reveals dual ancestry of Native Americans. *Nature* 505: 87–91. doi:10.1038/nature12736.

Renfrew, C. 1998. *Archaeology and language: The puzzle of Indo-European origins*. London: Pimlico.

Rootsi, S., L.A. Zhivotovsky, M. Baldovic, M. Kayser, I.A. Kutuev, R. Khusainova, M.A. Bermisheva, M. Gubina, S.A. Fedorova, A.M. Ilumae, E.K. Khusnutdinova, M.I. Voevoda, L. P. Osipova, M. Stoneking, A.A. Lin, V. Ferak, J. Parik, T. Kivisild, P.A. Underhill, and R. Villems. 2007. A counter-clockwise northern route of the Y-chromosome haplogroup N from Southeast Asia towards Europe. *European Journal of Human Genetics* 15: 204–211. doi:10.1038/sj.ejhg.5201748.

Shi, H., H. Zhong, Y. Peng, Y.L. Dong, X.B. Qi, F. Zhang, L.F. Liu, S.J. Tan, R.Z. Ma, C.J. Xiao, R.S. Wells, L. Jin, and B. Su. 2008. Y chromosome evidence of earliest modern human settlement in East Asia and multiple origins of Tibetan and Japanese populations. *BMC Biology* 6: 45. doi:10.1186/1741-7007-6-45.

Shou, W.H., E.F. Qiao, C.Y. Wei, Y.L. Dong, S.J. Tan, H. Shi, W.R. Tang, and C.J. Xiao. 2010. Y-chromosome distributions among populations in Northwest China identify significant contribution from Central Asian pastoralists and lesser influence of western Eurasians. *Journal of Human Genetics* 55: 314–322. doi:10.1038/jhg.2010.30.

Shubin, A.C. 1973. *Brief essay of ethnic history of the Evenks from Trans-Baikal region (XVIII–XX centries)*. Ulan-Ude: Buryat Publishing House. [in Russian].

Su, B., J. Xiao, P. Underhill, R. Deka, W. Zhang, J. Akey, W. Huang, D. Shen, D. Lu, J. Luo, J. Chu, J. Tan, P. Shen, R. Davis, L. Cavalli-Sforza, R. Chakraborty, M. Xiong, R. Du, P. Oefner, Z. Chen, and L. Jin. 1999. Y-Chromosome evidence for a northward migration of modern humans into Eastern Asia during the last Ice Age. *American Journal of Human Genetics* 65: 1718–1724. doi:10.1086/302680.

Tajima, A., M. Hayami, K. Tokunaga, T. Juji, M. Matsuo, S. Marzuki, K. Omoto, and S. Horai. 2004. Genetic origins of the Ainu inferred from combined DNA analyses of maternal and paternal lineages. *Journal of Human Genetics* 49: 187–193. doi:10.1007/s10038-004-0131-x.

Tambets, K., S. Rootsi, T. Kivisild, H. Help, P. Serk, E.L. Loogvali, H.V. Tolk, M. Reidla, E. Metspalu, L. Pliss, O. Balanovsky, A. Pshenichnov, E. Balanovska, M. Gubina, S. Zhadanov, L. Osipova, L. Damba, M. Voevoda, I. Kutuev, M. Bermisheva, E. Khusnutdinova, V. Gusar, E. Grechanina, J. Parik, E. Pennarun, C. Richard, A. Chaventre, J.P. Moisan, L. Barac, M. Pericic, P. Rudan, R. Terzic, I. Mikerezi, A. Krumina, V. Baumanis, S. Koziel, O. Rickards, G. F. De Stefano, N. Anagnou, K.I. Pappa, E. Michalodimitrakis, V. Ferak, S. Furedi, R. Komel, L. Beckman, and R. Villems. 2004. The western and eastern roots of the Saami—The story of genetic "outliers" told by mitochondrial DNA and Y chromosomes. *American Journal of Human Genetics* 74: 661–682. doi:10.1086/383203.

Tsydendambaev, T.B. 1972. *Buryatskiye istoricheskiye khroniki i rodoslovnye*. UlanUde: Buryat. knizh. izd.

Vainshtein, S. 1980. *Nomads South Siberia: The pastoral economies of Tuva*. Cambridge: Cambridge University Press.

Wells, R.S., N. Yuldasheva, R. Ruzibakiev, P.A. Underhill, I. Evseeva, J. Blue-Smith, L. Jin, B. Su, R. Pitchappan, S. Shanmugalakshmi, K. Balakrishnan, M. Read, N.M. Pearson, T. Zerjal, M.T. Webster, I. Zholoshvili, E. Jamarjashvili, S. Gambarov, B. Nikbin, A. Dostiev, O. Aknazarov, P. Zalloua, I. Tsoy, M. Kitaev, M. Mirrakhimov, A. Chariev, and W.F. Bodmer. 2001. The Eurasian heartland: A continental perspective on Y-chromosome diversity. *Proceedings of the National Academy of Sciences of the United States of America* 98: 10244–10249. doi:10.1073/pnas.171305098.

Xue, Y., T. Zerjal, W. Bao, S. Zhu, Q. Shu, J. Xu, R. Du, S. Fu, P. Li, M.E. Hurles, H. Yang, and C. Tyler-Smith. 2006. Male demography in East Asia: A north-south contrast in human population expansion times. *Genetics* 172: 2431–2439. doi:10.1534/genetics.105.054270.

Yan, S., H. Tachibana, L.H. Wei, G. Yu, S.Q. Wen, and C.C. Wang. 2015. Y chromosome of Aisin Gioro, the imperial house of the Qing dynasty. *Journal of Human Genetics* 60: 295–298. doi:10.1038/jhg.2015.28.

Yao, D., and J. Sun. 2012. From tribal confederacy to ethnic community: On historical changes in Manchu identity before the mid-Qing. In *Chinese schalors in inner Asia*, ed. X. Luo, and R. Covey. Bloomington, Indiana: Sinor Research Institute for Inner Asia Studies, Indiana University.

Zerjal, T., R.S. Wells, N. Yuldasheva, R. Ruzibakiev, and C. Tyler-Smith. 2002. A genetic landscape reshaped by recent events: Y-chromosomal insights into central Asia. *American Journal of Human Genetics* 71: 466–482. doi:10.1086/342096.

Zheng, L.H., H.M. Sun, J.W. Wang, S.L. Li, J. Bai, Y. Jin, Y. Yu, F. Chen, L. Jin, and S.B. Fu. 2009. Y chromosomal STR polymorphism in northern Chinese populations. *Biological Research* 42: 497–504. doi:10.4067/S0716-97602009000400011.

Zhong, H., H. Shi, X.B. Qi, C.J. Xiao, L. Jin, R.Z. Ma, and B. Su. 2010. Global distribution of Y-chromosome haplogroup C reveals the prehistoric migration routes of African exodus and early settlement in East Asia. *Journal of Human Genetics* 55: 428–435. doi:10.1038/jhg.2010.40.

Zhong, H., H. Shi, X.B. Qi, Z.Y. Duan, P.P. Tan, L. Jin, B. Su, and R.Z. Ma. 2011. Extended Y chromosome investigation suggests postglacial migrations of modern humans into East Asia via the northern route. *Molecular Biology and Evolution* 28: 717–727. doi:10.1093/molbev/msq247.

Zhou, R., D. Yang, H. Zhang, W. Yu, L. An, X. Wang, H. Li, J. Xu, and X. Xie. 2008. Origin and evolution of two Yugur sub-clans in Northwest China: A case study in paternal genetic landscape. *Annals of Human Biology* 35: 198–211. doi:10.1080/03014460801922927.

The Silk Road: Language and Population Admixture and Replacement

Dan Xu and Shaoqing Wen

1 Introduction

This paper investigates the (non-)correlation between languages and genes on the Silk Road. It is expected to provide a clear picture of human migration history between Central Asia and East Asia. It aims to study models of language formation and replacement on the Silk Road after the 13th century AD. Combining natural sciences and human sciences enables us to overcome the limits of traditional methodology in historical linguistics. In light of biological and archeological research results, where dating is based on concrete materials, our investigation will trace language ancestry on the Silk Road over the same timescales. Diachronic linguistics needs new approaches to go beyond its chronological limits.

The Silk Road is inhabited by different ethnic groups: Chinese (Han), Hui (Muslims), Santa (Dongxiang), Bao'an (Baonan), Monguor (Tu), Eastern Yugur (Yellow Uighur), Western Yugur, Salar, Amdo Tibetan Kazakh and Uyghur. This paper will take eight representative languages (Eastern Yugur, Tu, Dongxiang and Bao'an for Mongolic language group, and Uyghur, Kazakh, Western Yugur and Salar for Turkic group) in studying language admixture and replacement with a biological background. It will show that some languages are the result of admixture over several centuries, and others are newborn languages, like their populations: their

D. Xu (✉) · S. Wen
Institut National des Langues et Civilisations Orientales (INALCO),
63 Rue des Grands Moulins, Paris 75013, France
e-mail: xusongdan@gmail.com

D. Xu
CRLAO (CNRS), Paris, France

S. Wen
MOE Key Laboratory of Contemporary Anthropology, School of Life Sciences,
Fudan University, Shanghai 200433, People's Republic of China

D. Xu and H. Li (eds.), *Languages and Genes in Northwestern China and Adjacent Regions*, DOI 10.1007/978-981-10-4169-3_4

languages were completely replaced due to important historical migrations of their ancestors.

The field of linguistics was established in the 19th century. It is taken for granted that comparative studies of Indo-European languages are more advanced and mature thanks to tireless work by linguists. Their comparative method has been introduced to other language families.[1] If we take advantage of research results from other disciplines, we will have a wide-angle perspective from which we can observe many facets of a language. Molecular anthropology has seen significant development since the 1980s and provides linguistics and other domains with a powerful tool. Precise genetic dating will help us to better classify languages and language groups/families. Languages are carried by populations which are bearers of different genes. Comparing language distance based on ethnic genetic distance will help us to reconstruct different historical periods during which dispersing populations, bearers of diverse genes, also spread their languages. We must attempt to exploit new methods to improve our research and break down linguistic limits.

The paper will first present the distribution of languages and Y chromosomes in Northwest China, then analyze their (non)correlation. Two models of language formation/replacement will be studied based on these concrete data: (1) The Elite Dominance model, initially put forth by Renfrew (1987), will be revisited and refined; (2) The Culture Dominance model, proposed in this article, will complete the first model. Finally, preliminary conclusions will be given.

2 The Distribution of Languages and Y-Chromosomes in Northwest China

2.1 *Language Situation at the Basic Word Level*

Why are language-gene correlations often broken on the Silk Road? Based on existing historic, genetic and archeological work, we know today that populations living along the Silk Road formed at different periods from diverse ethnic sources. Every ethnic group has multiple origins. None of them come from just a single source. Their languages have undergone intense contact, admixture to different degrees, some of them were mixed and some others were replaced. The rate of change and of replacement is not homogenous. At different epochs, culture and religious factors have played an undeniable role in population and language admixture. Some languages were replaced by ones spoken by those who ruled their speakers, such as Mongolic languages on the Silk Road, but some others adopted another population's language due to cultural and religious factors, such as some

[1]But even today, there is not a strong consensus among linguists on the status of some language families (for example the Altaic family has been debated for decades), not to mention macro-families which are often even less certain.

Mongolian rulers like Chagatai and his descendants who underwent a Turkification in Central Asia.

The technique of glottochronology, a kind of linguistic clock proposed by Swadesh in the 1950s, is still widely used despite criticism from linguists. They sensibly rejected the view that the rate of change is even in every language. Nevertheless, linguistics researchers continue to use it in calculating language distances, keeping in mind that each language evolves with its own speed, and that each word has its own history. Unfortunately, linguists do not have other efficient means to quantify linguistic data, as do biologists who can use DNA sequences to estimate the separation of species or archeologists who can exploit radiocarbon to provide a fossil dating. Languages evolve at a much faster pace and the phonetics and semantics of words undergo uninterruptible change. A language could become unintelligible over a period of some decades due to phonetic and semantic changes. Even though the glottochronology method is not ideal, nor perfect, it is one of the appropriate ways to compare languages. A less rigorous method is always better than nothing. This paper also takes the list of 200 words established by Swadesh to study the relationship between languages on the Silk Road. In the past, cognate words between different languages have been widely studied in comparative studies. In this section we will first concentrate on the synchronic linguistic situation or the result of the phonetic evolution of the lexicon, not tracing back, for the moment, cognate words from a diachronic perspective. At this step, we will only account for phonetic differences. For example, "j-" in some languages is relative to "ʤ-" in other languages since they were cognate words and had the same source in the past, and "a-" in some languages is relative to "ha-" in other languages due to sound loss, or "-d-" in one language is connected to "-ʥ-" in another due to palatalization and so on. We count all synchronic phonetic differences as divergence in order to observe and compare their degrees of change. This method presents an advantage over traditional methods of calculating cognates. Synchronic differences are visible and objective, while diachronic differences and similarities are reconstructed differently from linguist to linguist. The criterion of cognate reconstruction could be subjective or biased. In the next section, we will also use cognate word statistics, limiting subjective reconstructions as much as possible. Actually these approaches are complementary to each other and both are needed to better understand language evolution. In the Turkic group we selected Uyghur, Tuva, Kazakh, Kirgiz, Western Yugur, Salar, and Tatar (Turkish is also used for comparison); in the Mongolic group we selected Mogolian, Dagur, Eastern Yugur, Tu (Monguor), Dongxiang (Santa) and Bao'an (Baonan) . Some languages of the Manchu-Tungusic group are also included as reference languages, including Manchu, Xibo (Xibe), Evenki, and Nanai.[2]

[2]Thanks to Saiyinjiya Caidengduoerji for digitizing Mongolic and Man-Tungusic language words, Barbara Kozhevina for Turkic language words.

After a preliminary comparative study in the Turkic group, it is noted that the lexical differences between seven languages (excluding contemporary Turkish for the moment) is not very large at the phonetic level. Concretely, in seven languages of the Turkic group within China, there exist on average less than three phonetic differences out of seven words for each entry in the 200 word list. As has been mentioned, every difference is accounted for even though these words are cognates coming from the same origin. The focus is to consider their divergence today. This means that in the Turkic group, more than half of the words have quasi-identical or similar pronunciations. In consequence, the result shows that in the Turkic group, the basic words in languages are quite stable after splitting, sharing more than 60% common words with quite similar pronunciation. When contemporary Turkish is added, the percentage is similar, keeping the same level. The literature on Turkic languages, their classifications and evolution is abundant. This paper has proposed another angle from which to observe the differences and divergence of these languages, being a complement to previous work on cognate words.

In contrast, languages in the Mongolic group present more variance. On average we find near four phonetic differences out of six words in every entry in the 200 word list. As result, the degree of similarity is about 40%. It has to be noticed that such statistics are indicative and not absolute. At least general tendencies can be seen through them. Manchu-Tungusic languages are not really spoken[3] on the Silk Road. They are conventionally classified with Turkic and Mongolic groups into the Altaic family. Their statistics serve here as a comparative reference. As has been expected, Manchu-Tungusic languages are closer to Mongolic languages but further from Turkic languages. Four Manchu-Tungusic languages are considered: Manchu, Xibo (or Xibe), Evenki and Nanai. Their phonetic difference is significant; on average, more than half of their words are divergent. Only 32% similarity is observed. Let us see the summary table.

Table 1 clearly suggests that a greater uniformity is observed in the Turkic group while it is much smaller in the Mongolic and Manchu-Tungusic groups. Even considering contemporary Turkish spoken outside of China, the divergence in Turkic languages is not as significant as in Mongolic languages.

In this section, 13 languages (excluding 4 Manchu-Tungusic languages and Turkish) on the Silk Road in China have been examined at a basic lexical level from a synchronic phonetic perspective. In Sect. 3, we will focus from diachronic point of view on eight representative languages which separately belong to Mongolic and Turkic groups on the Silk Road. The linguistic data will be broadened to include not only basic words but also frequent used vocabulary. Previous statistics completed by our own data will be presented and compared with genetic data.

[3]The Xibo people moved from the Northeast to the Northwest in 1764.

Table 1 Comparison of 200 basic words in Altaic languages spoken in China

Language group	Average difference	Variance	Similarity (%)
Turkic group (7 languages excluding Turkish)	2.84	1.98	60
Mongolic group (6 languages)	3.60	2.21	40
Manchu-Tungusic group (4 languages)	2.71	0.81	32

2.2 *Paternal Genetic Pattern in Northwest China*

Similar to intensive language contact among various linguistic families, especially between Sino-Tibetan and Altaic, population admixture had occurred at different times in history, leading to an extraordinary level of human diversity in Northwest China. Overall, four main paternal lineages, C, D, O and N, accounting for more than 90% of East Asian Y chromosomes, are also prevalent in Northwestern populations (Wang and Li 2013). However, Western Eurasia-specific Y chromosome haplogroups E, G, H, I, J, L, Q, R and T were found at relatively high frequencies in Northwest China, reflecting the recent gene flows from the west via the ancient Silk Road.

Here, to understand the genetic structure of the eight target populations, we genotyped 17 microsatellites by using a Y-filer kit (Applied Biosystems) and hierarchically typed Y chromosomes through seven panels of 100 SNPs as described in previous studies (Wang et al. 2014). A neighbor-joining (NJ) unrooted tree was then constructed based on frequencies of Y chromosome haplogroups using MEGA 5.1.

From this NJ tree, the overall clustering pattern of those populations was clearly displayed. Two Mongolic-speaking populations, Bao'an and Dongxiang from Gansu, formed a cluster with two representative Turkic-speaking populations, Uyghur and Salar. The remaining two Mongolic-speaking populations, Tu and Eastern Yugur, also contributed to this cluster. The Khazakhs and Western Yugur people, by contrast, have tended to be segregated away. Hence, at the population level, Turkic-speaking populations showed much larger genetic distances than Mongolic-speaking populations as viewed from their Y chromosomes.

Another noticeable feature from this analysis is that linguistic boundaries are often transgressed across the Altaic linguistic groups. Such a phenomenon is even more pronounced among Northwestern populations, where populations which have a common origin as recorded in historical records tend to cluster in the phylogeny. This observation is consistent with the history of Northwestern populations along the ancient Silk Road, where population migrations were substantial. In next section, we will present in detail the situation in each language and analyze the reasons for matches and mismatches (Fig. 1).

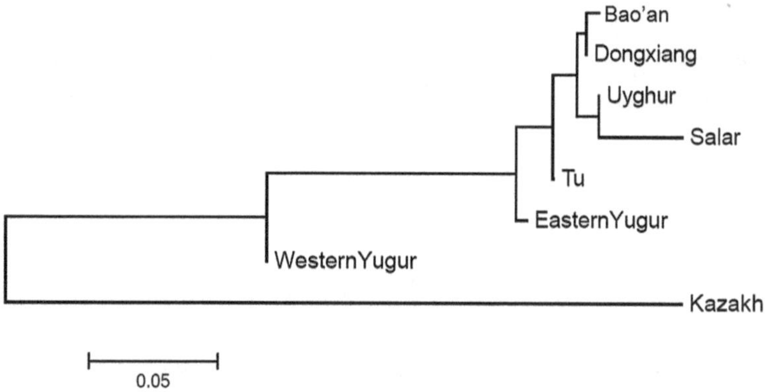

Fig. 1 Neighbor-joining trees of the Mongolic and Turkic-speaking populations based on frequencies of Y chromosome haplogroups

3 The Match and Mismatch of Two Datasets

An interdisciplinary approach will be used. In particular, historical, biological and archeological research results will be taken into account to evaluate the historic frame in which languages evolved. As has been mentioned, some languages and genes are not correlated on the Silk Road. We will first compare the linguistic and genetic data we have on the Mongolic group, then on the Turkic group within China.

3.1 Mongolic Languages and Paternal Genetic Correlations

The linguistic data is composed of the *Dictionary of Mongolic languages* compiled by Sun et al. (1990), articles by Chen (1990a, b), Menhedalai and Xing (1997), and our own statistics. Comparing Mongolian (Chakhar Mongolian in Inner Mongolia), Eastern Yugur, Dongxiang and Bao'an, it is seen that the percentage of cognate words to Mongolian is different and variable. Historians have shed light on populations on the Silk Road, and we now know that these four target peoples did not form in the same way. These groups each have their own characteristics concerning ethnic sources and tribal compositions. The Eastern Yugur and Tu languages correspond to Middle Mongolian, and share a significant proportion of cognates with contemporary Mongolian.

The Dongxiang and Bao'an languages however suggest another scenario. These Mongolic languages formed due to violent historical events. They are newly formed languages and most of their ancestors came from Central Asia and West Asia. Linguistic and genetic data are mismatched in these populations. The historian Liu (2003: 143) believes that at the beginning of the 13th century, a huge number of migrants were brought to China by Genghis Khan and his armies. There were young men forced to enroll in the army, as well as artisans of different handicrafts. This migration has left a mark on Chinese history, and even on East Asian history. It is impossible that this move did not leave any traces. These migrants were forced to learn Mongolian and today one finds few traces of Central Asian languages among these people. These Central Asians were Mongolized and their languages formed from 13th century Mongolian.

Eastern Yugur

According to the *Dictionary of Mongolic languages* compiled by Sun et al. (1990), cognate words between East Yugur and Mongolian make up 54%. This statistic is based on 2093 words. Our statistics show that the cognates make up 83% of the first 100 words, and 62% of the second hundred words. On average, 72.5% cognates are found among 200 words (Fig. 2).

Eighteen paternal lineages were determined from 45 individual eastern Yugur samples from Sunan Yugur Autonomous County in Gansu Province. The Yugur people are mainly comprised of two groups, Mongolic-speaking Eastern Yugur and Turkic-speaking Western Yugur. However, strong ethnic identity is shared between these two groups (Chen and Lei 1985; Zhaonasitu 1981a, b). In previous genetic investigations (Shou et al. 2010), it was inappropriate to employ sampling strategies that often ignored the individual's origin from Eastern Yugur or Western Yugur and thus failed to provide an insight into the relationship between language differentiation and population history. In this study, the major haplogroups C3*-M217, D1a*-N1+, N2-, D3a-P47 and J-M304 are prevalent in Eastern Yugur. Haplogroup C3*-M217, which occurs at high frequencies in Mongolic-speaking populations (Di Cristofaro et al. 2013; Kharkova et al. 2014; Malyarchuk et al. 2010; Zerjal et al. 2003; Zhong et al. 2010), is also observed at a high frequency in Eastern Yugur (14.3%), suggesting a genetic link between Eastern Yugur and Mongolian populations. Typical paternal markers of Tibetan and Qiang populations (Shi et al. 2008), D1-M15 and D3-P47, are also found with high frequency in Eastern Yugur. Most D1-M15 and D3-P47 haplotypes in Yugur populations are also found in surrounding populations in Gansu (such as Hui and Han) and in Tibetans from Qinghai province, exhibiting a profound influence from Tibetan populations. It is particularly noteworthy that West Eurasian haplogroup J-M304 (Zhong et al. 2011) is detected at considerable frequencies in Eastern Yugur. One J-M304 haplotype is

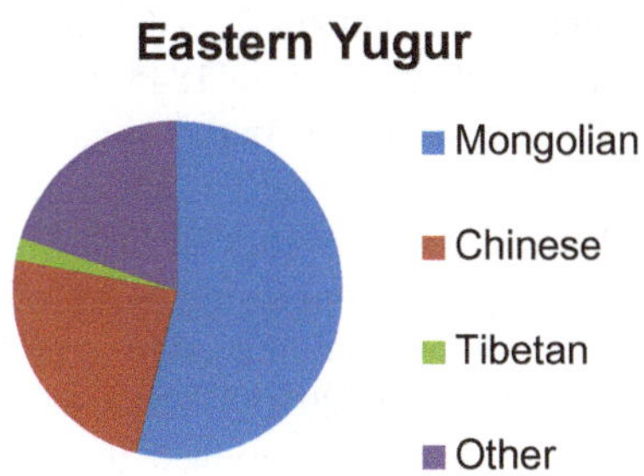

Fig. 2 Different sources of the Eastern Yugur language (based on Sun et al. 1990)

Fig. 3 Observed paternal lineages in Eastern Yugur

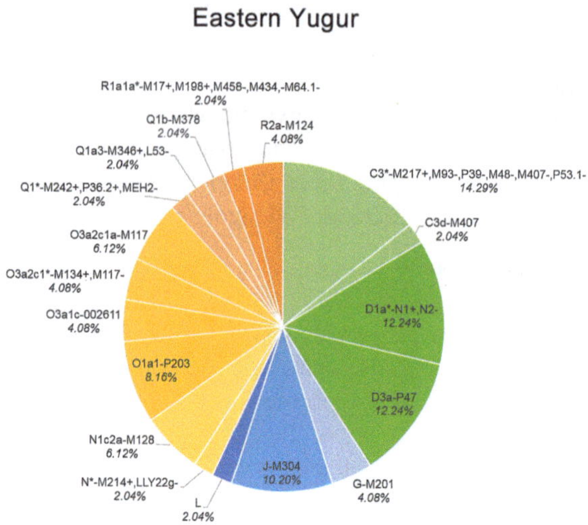

shared between Eastern Yugur, Uyghur and Hui in Gansu province, implying that they have experienced common historical events (Fig. 3).

Tu (Monguor)

The origin of Tu has been discussed by historians and linguists (Zhou 2004; Li 2008; Qie 2009 among others). The most popular idea is that the Tu people constitute one of the branches of the Mongols and their origin is from Xianbei. The core ancestors of Tu were Tuyuhun khan and his offspring, Tyuhun came from Murong tribes. During the initial formation, Qiang, Tibetan and Chinese people joined this clan. After the disintegration of the Tuyuhun Kingdom (4–7th centuries), some populations were Tibetanized and others Sinicized. The genetic data also suggests that the contribution from Central Asia is not negligible. Linguistic data shows that, as Eastern Yugur, the Tu language shares the same proportion of cognates with Mongolian. Specialists think that Tu is very similar to 13th century Mongolian (Zhaonasitu 1981a; Li 2008). Mongolian vocabulary is shown to make up a major portion in Sun et al. (1990) with a significant percentage of Chinese loans. Other sources are not significant in number. Please see the following figures. In our statistics, in the 100 word list, Tu share cognates with Mongolian at a percentage of 78% while in the second 100 word list, it attains 65%. On average, cognates account for 71.5%. The following figure is based on Sun et al. (1990), with statistics based on 1845 words (Fig. 4).

Twenty-four paternal lineages were determined from the 121 individual Tu samples from Huzhu Tu Autonomous County in Qinghai Province. Haplogroups R1a1a-M17, D1-M15, O3a2c1a-M117, O3a1c-002611 were the most frequent lineages, together comprising 44.6% of the Tu people's paternal gene pool. Haplogroup R1a1a-M17 is predominant in some Turkic-speaking populations (Di Cristofaro et al. 2013; Shou et al. 2010; Wells et al. 2001) and appears with relatively high frequency in Tu people. As mentioned above, haplogroups D1-M15 and D3a-P47, associated

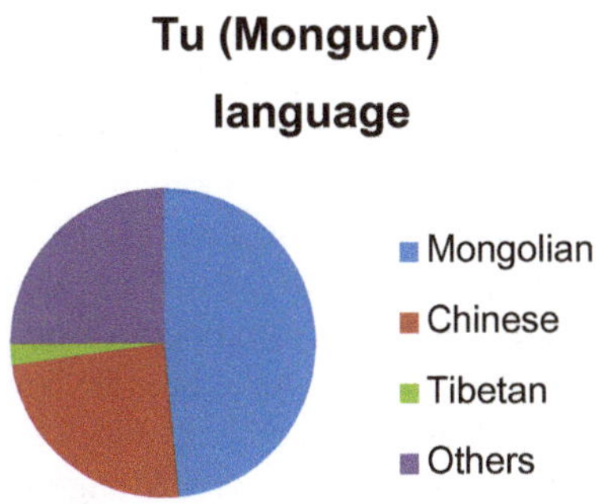

Fig. 4 Different sources of the Tu language (based on Sun et al. 1990)

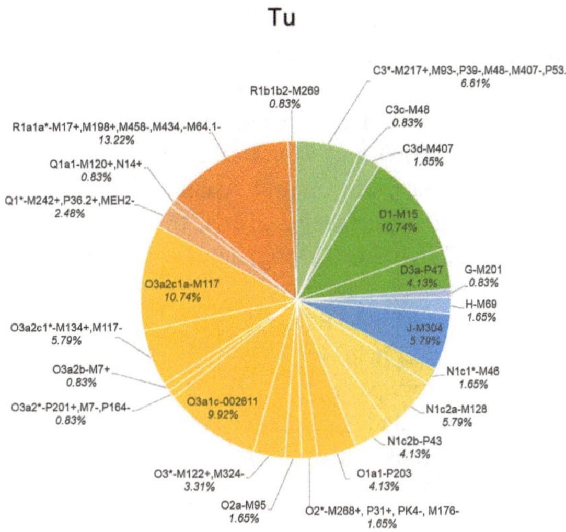

Fig. 5 Observed paternal lineages in Tu

with Tibeto-Burman populations (Shi et al. 2008), are also observed at a high frequency and moderate frequency in Tu (10.74 and 4.13%, respectively). Main sublineages of O3-M122, O3a2c1a-M117, O3a1c-002611, accounting for 20.7% of the Tu samples, which are predominant in Han and Hui populations but are rare or absent in Mongolic and Turkic populations (Di Cristofaro et al. 2013; Shou et al. 2010; Wells et al. 2001; Wen et al. 2004). Hence these lineages can be treated as genetic influences from Han and Hui populations in the same region. Notably, haplogroup C3*-M217, as well as C3c-M48 and C3d-M407, is the common paternal lineage in Mongolic-speaking populations (Di Cristofaro et al. 2013; Kharkova et al. 2014; Malyarchuk et al. 2010; Zerjal et al. 2003; Zhong et al. 2010), which are also found at moderate or relatively low levels in the Tu people, indicating the complicated genetic connection between Tu and Mongolian populations (Fig. 5).

Dongxiang

The origin of the Dongxiang people is clear. At least more than half (unpublished statistics from Fudan's laboratory) of the population came from Central Asia (cf also Shou et al. 2010). As has been mentioned, this language formed during the

14th century due to the large migration after the conquest by Genghis Khan of Central Asia in the 13th century. The following chart is based on our research published in 2013 showing that the Dongxiang vocabulary (based on 10994 words) has Mongolian as its main source, keeping only 5.65% of the parent language's vocabulary. Chinese loan words make up around 35%. Today, the Dongxiang language is considered to be a Mongolian variety; actually it was a replaced language, i.e. the ancestral populations might have spoken other languages of Central Asia and Western Asia, but they were forced to change their mother tongue by the ruler's language in order to survive. As for the first 100 basic words, Dongxiang has 70% cognate words with Mongolian, and in the second hundred words, the percentage is 48%. On average, 59% of words cognate with Mongolian can be found on the list of 200 words. The linguistic situation is quite similar to Bao'an, another replaced language on the Silk Road. The following graph is based on 10994 words (Fig. 6).

In our previous study, we studied Y-chromosomal data drawn from the literature (Wen et al. 2013) and found that the Dongxiang people did not descend from Mongolians, but from Central Asian and Western Asian ethnic groups that spoke Persian or Turkic languages. Here, twenty-five paternal lineages were determined from the 107 individual Dongxiang samples from Dongxiang Autonomous County in Gansu Province. Relatively high frequencies of the western Y chromosomal haplogroups J-M304, R1a1a-M17 and R2a-M124 in Dongxiang people further strengthen our conclusion that the Dongxiang people are much closer to Central Asian ethnic groups than to the other Mongolians. Additional admixture, in the presence of low and moderate frequencies of the typical East Asian haplogroups C, D, N and O, took place primarily on their migration route or during subsequent settlement in Northwest China (Fig. 7).

Bao'an

Like Dongxiang, the genes of Bao'an populations came from Central Asian people, but linguistically, their language belongs to the Mongolic language group. Chen studies (1990b: 32) indicate that Bao'an should be divided into two dialects, one in Qinghai (Nianduhu) and one in Gansu (Ganhetan). These two dialects show a different rate of change, conditioned by their geographic separation and different religious beliefs. The statistics by Chen (1990a: 17) are based on 3596 words in Nianduhu Bao'an and 3624 in Ganhetan Bao'an. According to him, 28.70% of Mongolian cognate words are found in Nianduhu and 28.12% in Ganhetan. In the

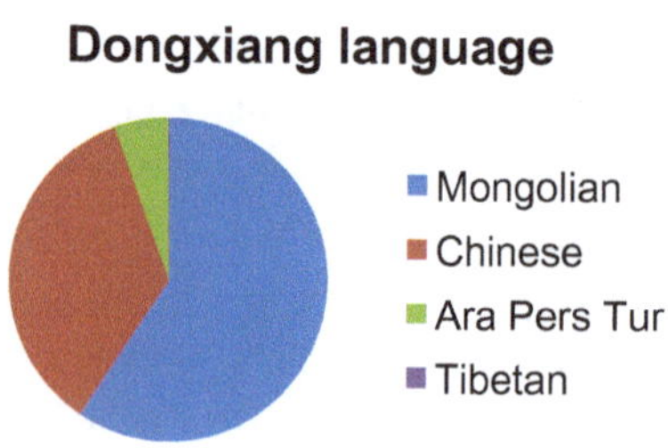

Fig. 6 Different sources of the Dongxiang language (based on Dan Xu 2014)

Fig. 7 Observed paternal lineages in Dongxiang

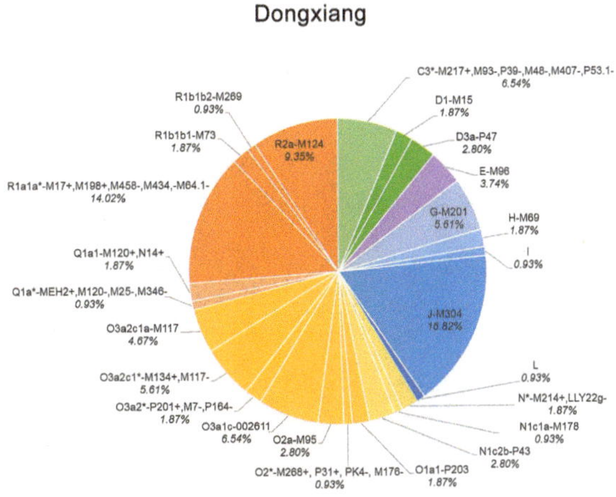

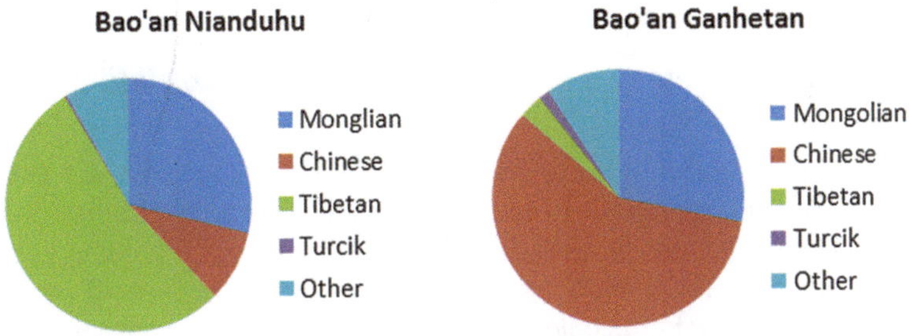

Fig. 8 Comparison between two Bao'an dialects (based on Cheng Naixiong 1990a)

basic vocabulary, we count 71% cognates with Mongolian in the first 100 word list and 47% cognates in the second 100 word list. In consequence, 59% cognate words with Mongolian are seen on average for 200 words. This result is almost identical with Dongxiang.

Chen (1990a: 17) provides interesting comparative studies. He remarks that in the two dialects of Bao'an, Nianduhu has borrowed 53.62% of words from Amdo Tibetan and Ganhetan has borrowed 58.11% of loan words from Chinese, but the consequence is different. He thinks that Bao'an in Nianduhu has maintained its syntax relatively well despite heavy borrowings while Bao'an in Ganhetan began to change its syntax due to intense language contact (Fig. 8).

Twenty-one paternal lineages were determined from the 64 individual Bao'an samples from Jishishan Bao'an, Dongxiang and Salar Autonomous County in Gansu Province. Three dominant lineages of the Bao'an paternal gene pool were identified based on their putative origin: West Eurasian (J-M304), Sino-Tibetan (O3a2c1a-M117) and Mongolian (C3*-M217). This result is in agreement with the hypothesis of their ancient presence in the West Eurasia and their subsequent population admixture with Sino-Tibetan and Mongolian populations in Northwest China (Fig. 9).

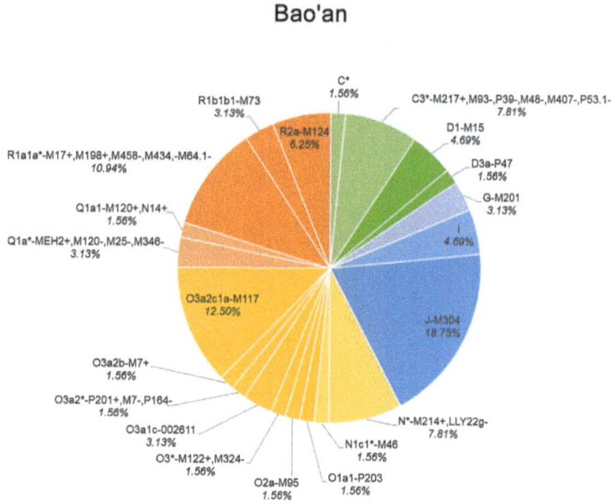

Fig. 9 Observed paternal lineages in Bao'an

3.2 *Turkic Languages and Paternal Genetic Correlations*

The four languages in the Turkic group, Uyghur, Western Yugur, Kazakh and Salar formed at different periods and from different clans, except Uyghur and Western Yugur which are thought to be from the same ancestral tribes. According to historic documents, after the fall of the Uyghur Khanate which was defeated by Yenisei Kirghiz in 840, the Uyghur people were divided into three groups dispersing from valleys of the Selenga River and the Orkhon River. One group established the Kara-Khanid dynasty (10–13th centuries) between today's Xinjiang and the Pamirs in Central Asia. It ended with Genghis Khan's conquest toward the West. The second group became the Uyghur of Gaochang (Xingjiang, 10–13th centuries), which also ended with Mongol armies headed by Genghis Khan. These populations are believed to be part of the ancestors of modern Uyghur in Xingjiang. Finally the third group was the Hexi Uyghur, also called Ganzhou Uyghur (900–1036). Their rulers were overthrown by Li Yuanhao, emperor of Tangut. These peoples are identified as the forefathers of the Western Yugur. Kazakh people were composed mainly of Mongolian populations (see genetic analysis) which underwent a Turkification. Salar people came from Central Asia and their origin is clear since research from different domains such as history, anthropology, linguistics and genetics has converged without exception. During the formation of these peoples, other ethnic groups joined them forming populations with diverse origins. In these four languages, contemporary Uyghur and Kazakh are the best preserved Turkic language in China. Chinese loan words are present at the lowest level in these two languages, while in Western Yugur and Salar, Chinese borrowings at the lexical level show a significant percentage. The linguistic data is mainly based on the *Dictionary of Turkic languages in China* by Chen et al. (1990), supplemented with published documents and our own statistics. The dictionary compiled by Chen et al.

is the most complete dictionary of contemporary Turkic languages in China. Let us see concrete data.

Uyghur

As mentioned earlier, due to their historical and cultural background, Uyghurs have been less influenced by Sinitic languages. Chinese loan words only make up around 3.19% in Uyghur. Its cognate words with other Turkic languages are significant, with 17.74% words of Arabic origin and 10.72% Persian words. As we know, Uyghurs are believed to be one of the three branches that came from Old Uyghurs who migrated from valleys of the Selenga River and the Orkhon River to Xinjiang after the fall of their khanate. Xinjiang has always been a meeting place of West with East. At this site, Tocharian, Sogdian and other western languages were spoken and then extinguished due to climate conditions and cultural and religious conflicts. Old Persian and Arabic, Old Chinese and other languages had also left traces in Uyghur languages and dialects over the centuries. Modern Chinese and Russian have also influenced Uyghur but the impacts seem to be much smaller than from Arabic and Persian. These two languages can be considered as traces of language contact in an earlier stratum. The following figure is based on 4075 words (Fig. 10).

The Uyghur people, which account for about half of the total population of Xinjiang, are a population presenting a typical admixture of Eastern and Western anthropometric traits. In this article, twenty-seven paternal lineages were determined from the 134 individual Uyghur samples from Turpan City. As predicted, on the one hand, Central-South Asia and West Eurasia related haplogroups R1a1a-M17 and J-M304 have also been detected at considerable frequencies, especially R1a1a-M17, which contributes 19.83% of Uyghur; on the other hand, relatively high frequencies of North Asia and East Asia related haplogroups C3*-M217 and O3a2c1*-M134 +, M117- were observed in Uyghur populations. Our result clearly indicates a typical genetic admixture pattern in the Uyghur population with ancestries from both eastern Eurasia and western Eurasia (Fig. 11).

Western Yugur

Here the linguistic data in Eastern Yugur is considered again in comparison with Western Yugur. It has been recognized that Eastern Yugur and Western Yugur

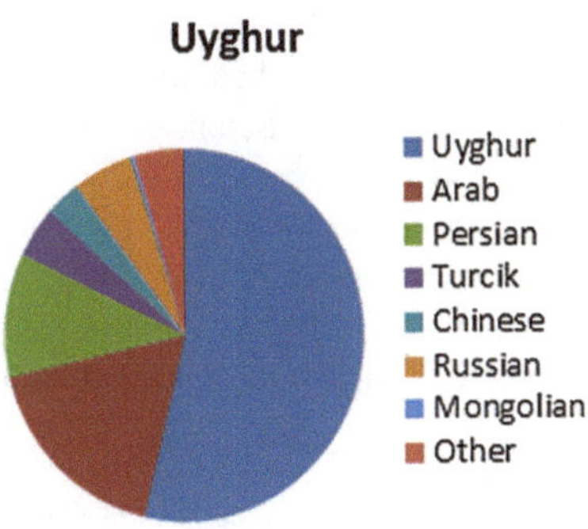

Fig. 10 Different sources of the Uyghur language (based on Chen et al. 1990)

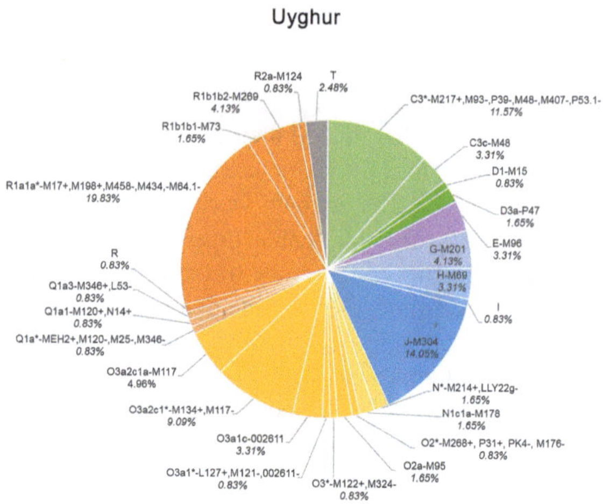

Fig. 11 Observed paternal lineages in Uyghur

belong to two subgroups (Mongolian and Turkic) of one language family, Altaic. In spite of their centuries-long union, their languages remain independent and even today they cannot communicate if one is not bilingual.[4] The populations speaking these two languages are located in the vast grasslands of southern Gansu, known as Sunan. Comparing these two following Figures, it is shown that WY is heavily influenced by Chinese at the lexical level (38%). The basis of statistics for WY is 3404 words while for EY we have 2093 words. Despite these significant lexical borrowings from Chinese, it seems that the syntax of WY has not been affected. Based on 851 frequent and comparable words, WY and EY share 13.74% common words. Chinese loanwords make up almost 19% in WY while they only present 9% in EY (Fig. 12).

In total, 54 WY samples were collected from Sunan Yugur Autonomous County. Haplogroups C3*-M217, O3a2c1a-M117 and Q1a*-MEH2+, M120-, M25-, M346- were the most frequent lineages in WY. In comparison of their haplogroup frequencies, EY and WY have considerable differences. Haplogroups D3a-P47 and O1a1-P203 was significantly more frequent in EY (12.24% and 8.16%, respectively) than in WY (both absent). Additionally, C3*-M217 and Q1a2a*-L53+, M3- was significantly more frequent in WY (41.18%) than in EY. Notably, Haplogroup Q1a2a*-L53+, M3- has so far only been found in Altain, Hui and Tuvan (Dulik et al. 2012 and unpublished data by the Laboratory of Contemporary Anthropology, School of Life Sciences, Fudan University). Altain and Tuvan are two Turkic-speaking populations in South Siberia. This lineage represented the close genetic relationship of the Yugur population with Tuvan and Altain in South Siberia. Interestingly, three of six Q1a2a*-L53+, M3- samples share the same family name "Yaghlaqar" (Yang in Chinese, see Sect. 4.1). This family name is inherited from the royal family of the ancient Uyghur Khanate (Li 2010; Yang 2003; Zhang 1991).

[4]Their language of communication is the Chinese language.

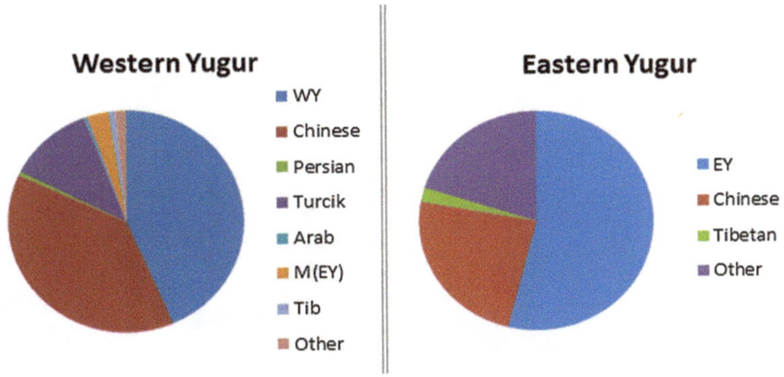

Fig. 12 Comparison between WY and EY (based on Chen et al. 1990; Sun et al. 1990)

Fig. 13 Observed paternal lineages in Western Yugur

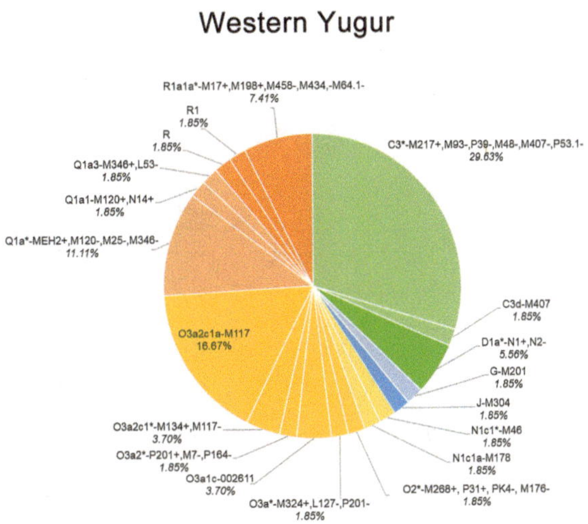

The genetic signal we observed here clearly shows a genetic tie between ancient Uygur people and present-day Tuvan and Altain. Therefore, although most haplogroups are shared between these two groups, strong paternal differentiation can also be observed between Turkic Yugur and Mongolic Yugur (Fig. 13).

Kazakh

According to historic records, Kazakh people constitute a combination of Mongols and Kazakh people who later formed a community of Turkic tribes. Due to Islamic religion and culture, a significant number of Mongolic tribes, often headed by Genghis Khan's offspring, joined Kazakh clans. The process of Turkification lasted 150 years (Lin and Gao 1994). It is amazing to observe that this Turkification was so complete that these converted Mongol tribes completely absorbed the Turkic language. To a certain extent, one can say that the mother tongue of these Mongols

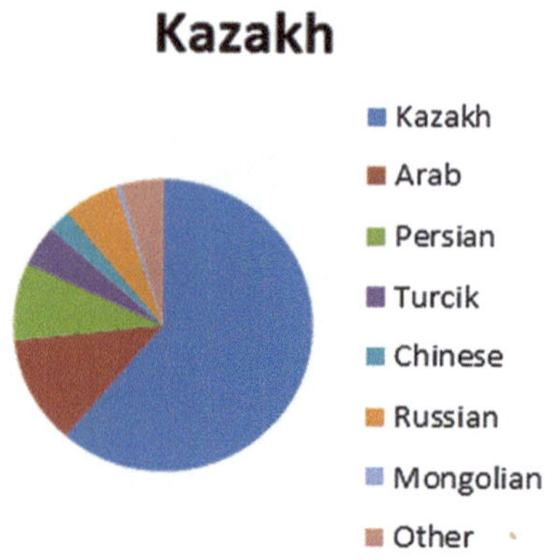

Fig. 14 Different sources of the Kazakh language (based on Chen et al. 1990)

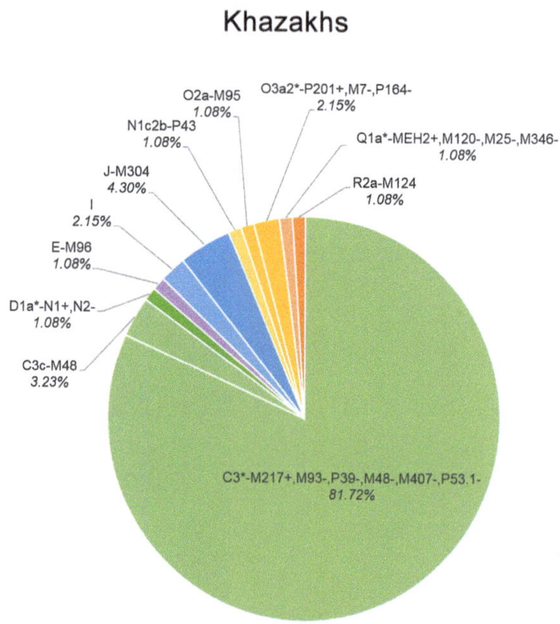

Fig. 15 Observed paternal lineages in Kazakh

was replaced by a Turkic language. As in modern Uyghur, Chinese loan words in the Kazakh language are almost insignificant, while Arabic and Persian words account for nearly 21% (Fig. 14).

Eleven paternal lineages were determined from 93 individual Kazakh samples from Aksai Kazakh Autonomous County in Gansu Province. This population presented the lower haplogroup and haplotype diversity values compared to the other studied populations, as they were mainly from a part of Kerey tribe that experienced a series of founder effects or strong bottlenecks when emigrating from Xinjiang Province to Gansu Province (Xie and Wang 2009). Haplogroup C3*-M217 comprises an overwhelming majority of Gansu Kazakh people (81.72%), reflecting the complex history of interaction between Turkic-speaking populations and Mongolic-speaking populations (Fig. 15).

Salar

Historians such as Mi (1981) think that Salars were descendants of Salor clans which belonged to Oghuz tribes. It is believed that they were brought into China by Genghis Khan from Samarkand after his victory in Central Asia. Oral legends say that these populations settled in Qinghai after a long travel led by two brothers who could not stand local repression of their family. Historical records tell us that Salars had helped Genghis Khan in beating the Tangut kingdom which fell in 1227 (see Mi 1981). Whatever the reason for their movement from Central Asia to Xunhua in Qinghai, they were probably recruited as conscripted troops like the Santa (today called Dongxiang) and Bao'an populations. Unlike Uyghur and Kazakh, Arabic and Persian sourced words only make up 5.3% at a basis of 3147 words while Chinese loanwords reach almost 32%, comparable to the lexical borrowing level of Western Yugur (Fig. 16).

Twenty paternal lineages were determined from the 134 individual Salar samples from Xunhua Salar Autonomous County in Gansu Province. Similar to the

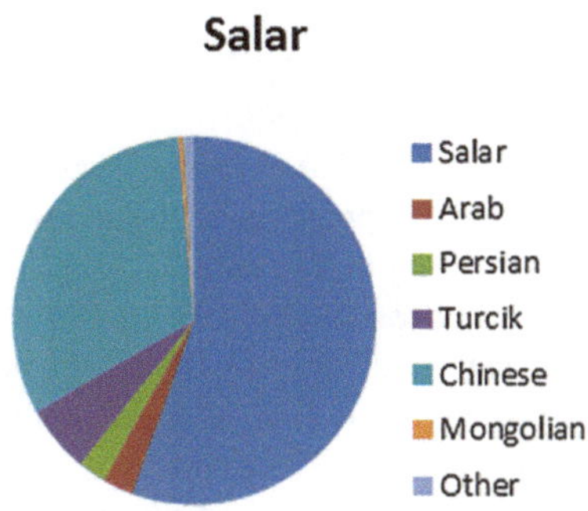

Fig. 16 Different sources of the Salar language (based on Chen Zongzhen et al. 1990)

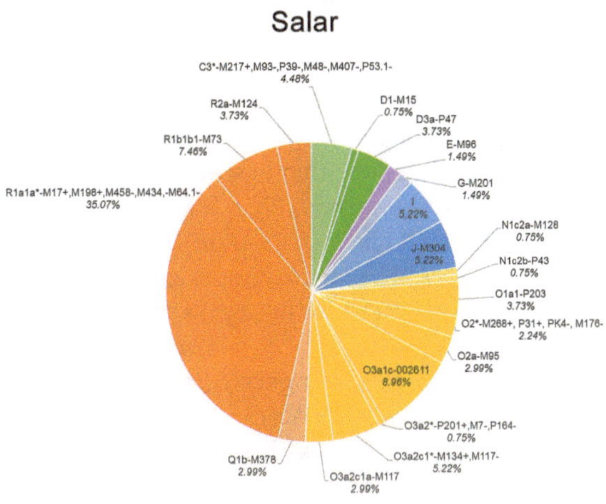

Fig. 17 Observed paternal lineages in Salar

Y-chromosomal lineage C3*-M217 in Gansu Kazakh people, the Central Asian specific Y-chromosomal lineages R1a1a*-M17 is observed at extremely high frequency in Salar people (35.07%). The presence of haplogroups C, D, N, O and Q at lower frequency is due to local population admixture, because haplotype sharing among these populations exists, which is consistent with historical records about the formation of the Salar population (Fig. 17).

4 Two Models of Language Replacement on the Silk Road

Grounded on our eight linguistic and genetic samples belonging to Mongolic and Turkic groups, we will observe admixture and replacement of these languages on the Silk Road. It is certain that different models of language replacement exist and language replacement can be provoked by numerous reasons. Here we will focus on two main models from our point of view, *Elite Dominance* model and *Cultural Dominance* model.

4.1 Elite Dominance Model

The Elite Dominance model was first proposed by Renfrew (1987) in a language replacement process. It assumes that newcomers bring natives into subjection causing language change. Language coexistence may last a time and a bilingual situation subsists at the beginning stage. One possible result is that the indigenous language is replaced by that of the newcomers after a bilingual period. According to Renfrew's model, new dominant peoples possess an organized society, and/or advanced military technologies such as horse riding, wheel fabrication and so on. These small groups which have technical and political advantages over larger resident populations, will have the chance to dominate the local residents. Renfrew took Proto-Europeans as a reference from an archeological perspective.

Here we use the *Elite Dominance model*, slightly modifying it to apply to situations on the Silk Road. Within this model, two situations can be considered or refined: (1) a group with few members, generally a ruler group or military conquerors, force a larger group to speak the dominant group's language. We will call these groups RULER GROUPS; (2) a few clans which occupy a higher social position due to their clan founder status or royal offspring origin, unify scattered clans from different sources. The language spoken by the core clans is venerated as common language and followed by other less influenced tribes. We will call these groups LEADER GROUPS.

In our target region, Dongxiang and Bao'an are two typical samples in which the language formation or replacement can be explained by a RULER GROUP i.e. the first *Elite Dominance* model. As has been mentioned in previous sections, Dongxiang and Bao'an people have their main ancestral sources in Central Asia. Their core ancestors were brought by Genghis Khan and his army to China. They were forced to settle in a region corresponding to today's borders between Gansu and Qinghai to participate in military activities or produce goods for the military. Small groups of Mongolian officers governed larger immigrant populations who likely spoke different languages or dialects of their homelands. One can imagine that at the beginning they were forced to learn Mongolian taking it as an official language to communicate one to each other.

Comparing genetic and linguistic datasets shows that languages and genes present a disagreement in Dongxiang and Bao'an. These comparative studies lead us to assume that the original languages of these populations were replaced in the past. More concretely, these peoples originated after the 13th century and their languages were newly created. Historical documents suggest that Dongxiang and Bao'an formed around the 14th century. This partly illuminates why the western branch of the Mongolic language group clearly shows different properties which are unique with respect to other Mongolic languages.

Now let us observe the LEADER GROUP situation, representing another case of the *Elite Dominance* model. In this case, populations are not forced to speak the language of dominant groups, but rather deliberately follow the tribe leaders which form core clans, and are respected by different smaller tribes. They joined the core tribes in periods of important events (military or political). This is the case of Yugur people. These clans headed by two leader families are composed of two groups: Western Yugur and Eastern Yugur. Western Yugur belongs to the Turkic language group and Eastern Yugur to the Mongolic language group. Yugur populations were nomads in the past and some of them have kept this lifestyle today. They are formed by different clans or families, with more than 14,000 persons nowadays, being composed of around fifty clans or families which each inherited their ancestral tribe name. Fifty Yugur family names reveal quite diverse sources representing each Yugur clan and allow us to trace back the multiple origins of Yugur populations embedded into two main groups, Western Yugur and Eastern Yugur. The case of Yugur clearly shows that diverse ethnic people were incorporated into these two famous clans speaking languages of these two families.

As has been mentioned in Sect. 3.2, Western Yugur and Uyghur may come from common ancestors who split in 840 after their Khanate fell due to Yenisei Kirghiz. Due to their different religious beliefs, some Old Uyghurs escaped from Xingjiang and settled in Gansu becoming Western Yugur. Among them, one family is famous for being one the founders of the Old Uyghur khanate. This clan's name is Yaklagar, with a Sinicized name *Yang* today. Actually, the name is already attested in Suji inscriptions and Terkhin inscriptions, thought to be Old Turcik from the 8th century. This name is also found in historic documents in Chinese such as *Song Shi* (Annals of Song, around 14th century). With genetic data, we observe that their ethnic sources are diverse, unifying multiple people coming from Turkic, Mongolic, Tibetan and other smaller tribes. We suppose that those people, who had joined the Yaklagar clan, must have learned the Turkic language for communication.

Another famous clan, Anjang, is the leader of the Eastern Yugur. Since the emperor of the Ming Dynasty (1368–1644) designated Buyan Tömöl as

Andingwang (King of maintaining stability), the Anjang clan has officially been considered the leader clan of the Yugur (Western and Eastern). The historian Gao (2000: 134–136) supposes that this family consists of Genghis Khan's descendants. The genetic data tells us that ethnic sources of Eastern Yugur are as diverse as Western Yugur. From a genetic perspective, C*-M217+ is believed (Zerjal et al. 2003; Abilev et al. 2012) to be the characteristic lineage from Genghis Khan's clan. It is found in both Eastern and Western Yugur people. This data may correspond to the fact that a governor from the Anjang family was sent to every tribe as leader since the beginning of the Ming Dynasty around the 14th century. This suggests the same scenario within which different tribes or clans were attracted by this key family and learned Mongolian, the source language of Eastern Yugur.

In the *Elite Dominance* model, as has been seen, the RULER GROUP forces the subjected people to speak the dominators' language, while the LEADER GROUP possesses a centripetal force to attract diverse populations to learn the leader tribes' languages.

4.2 Cultural Dominance Model

In the present work, a second model will be presented in the process of language formation and replacement: the *Cultural Dominance* model. In this model, populations adopting the culture and religion of another community are assimilated into a different ethnic group. This can happen to a group with a significant populations size, or to a small group of dominators.

Yugur is an interesting example. One group of Yugur residing in Huangnipu (Jiuquan county of Gansu province) has been completely Sinicized, perhaps since the Qing Dynasty.[5] This group of around 1000 people changed its lifestyle from nomadic to agrarian. Influenced by Chinese culture and language, these populations totally adopted the Chinese language and culture and do not speak Western Yugur any more. Geographically they are located very close to Jiuquan City (in Jiuquan County, Gansu) separated from other Yugurs who are still mainly nomadic. The Chinese language and cultural influences are much stronger than those exerted on the vast grassland in the south of Gansu. Their nomadic lifestyle has prevented Yugur people from losing their culture and language while an agrarian lifestyle caused the identity loss of other Yugur. This is one of the results of the *Cultural Dominance* model.

This also happened to a significant part of Kazakh populations. Haplogroup C-M130 is very frequent in Mongolian people, but occupies a high percentage (by different papers' statistics) in Kazakh populations speaking the Turkic language. Historic documents show us that Kazakh people are in fact mixed with Mongolian

[5]Saliyanyu (2000: 592) indicates that Yaklagar tribe-head-system was abolished by the Qing government in Huangnipu.

people due to Genghis Khan's descendants. Chagatai (the second son of Genghis Khan) and his offspring were rulers, but were surrounded by Central Asian populations which followed Islam. Over less than two centuries, these Mongolian rulers and their tribes underwent a Turkification and began to speak Turkic languages. This language replacement was due to their change of religious belief. This assimilation by Mongolic groups was voluntary and deliberate, due to cultural and religious factors. This time, the dominant culture came from dominated people, but the dominators, being converted into a new cultural system, accepted with their own volition the religion of dominated peoples. The bridge leading them to accomplish this change was the Turkic language.

The other famous example of language replacement caused by the *Cultural Dominance* model is the Manchu. The Manchurians were rulers in China from 1616 to 1911. The Manchu language is today almost extinct. This language replacement has been studied by scholars such as Ji (2004, 2005) who indicates three stages in which Manchu gradually declined and was replaced. Manchu was spoken alongside Mandarin in Beijing at the beginning of the 18th century, but the bilingual situation changed to monolingual in the 19th century. Finally Manchu was no longer spoken even by descendants of Manchu populations. This case is another example in which a RULER GROUP accepted the culture of foreign populations dominated by it.

Here two models are presented with concrete examples. Except for the last case with Manchu, other cited examples are all attested on the Silk Road. It is possible that language replacement occurred more than once for some languages and for some people.

5 Discussion

In this article, we have compared two sets of data, linguistic and genetic in a biological sense, from populations on the Silk Road. Our analysis focused on eight languages and populations belonging to Mongolic and Turkic groups. It has shown that languages and genes often do not correlate on the Silk Road due to multiple factors. It has been assumed that the Western branch of the Mongolic group often reveals particular properties in their language due to important historical events. This branch indeed has a special status on the Silk Road since these languages were newly formed from speakers of different languages. Dongxiang, Bao'an, and a large part of Kazakh people present instances of language replacement. But the reasons for replacement are quite distinct. One can be explained by the *Elite Dominance* model, as is the case for Dongxiang and Bao'an which are newborn or replaced languages which formed, around 14th century and the other by the *Cultural Dominance* model, which is the case for Kazakh which formed when a majority of Mongolic groups underwent Turkification around the 13 and 14th centuries (see Lin and Gao 1994: 226–227). Remember that the cases of Dongxiang and Bao'an belong to the first situation, i.e. the RULER GROUP of the *Elite Dominance* model, in which dominated populations were forced to change their language.

Yugur populations have been divided into two groups, Western Yugur and Eastern Yugur. It has been shown that both groups had multiple source clans. Different ethnicities have contributed to their formation. Concretely, among Eastern Yugurs, Tibetan populations which have joined Mongolic clans in the past were Mongolized, also including an important part of Han populations. Western Yugur populations, speakers of Turkic languages, were significantly enlarged by Mongolic clans at different periods. This corresponds well to historic documents (see Lin and Gao 1994: 258) which reveal that some Mongolic clans joined Sari Uyghurs at the beginning of the Ming Dynasty (1368–1644). Yugur populations clearly reflect the *Elite Dominance* model in which the second situation, i.e. a LEADER GROUP, played a key role in their language choice. Yugurs in Huangnipu, who have been Sinicized, have followed the *Cultural Dominance* model.

It is evident that language formation and replacement can be provoked by multiple factors and reasons. Explanations and analysis provided by this paper are tentative rather than rules. Our interdisciplinary approach attempts to take advantage of research results from different domains, in particular linguistics and molecular biology, to provide a description of a historical scenario which should be closer and more faithful to reality.

References

Abilev, S., B. Malyarchuk, M. Derenko, M. Wozniak, T. Grzybowski, and I. Zakharov. 2012. The Y-chromosome C3* star-cluster attributed to Genghis Khan's descendants is present at high frequency in the Kerey clan from Kazakhstan. *Human Biology* 84: 79–89.

Chen, Naixiong. 1990a. Tracing the evolution of Bao'an. *Minzu yuwen* [Non-Han languages] 3: 16–25.

Chen, Naixiong 1990b. Tracing the evolution of Bao'an (continuation). *Minzu yuwen* [Non-Han languages] 4: 42–48.

Chen, Zongzhen, et al. 1990. *A Lexicon of Turkish languages in China*. Beijing: Minzu chubanshe.

Chen, Z., and X. Lei. 1985. *Brief records of West Yugur language*. Beijing: Nationalities Publishing House.

Di Cristofaro, J., E. Pennarun, S. Mazieres, N.M. Myres, A.A. Lin, S.A. Temori, M. Metspalu, E. Metspalu, M. Witzel, R.J. King, P.A. Underhill, R. Villems, and J. Chiaroni. 2013. Afghan Hindu Kush: Where Eurasian sub-continent gene flows converge. *PLoS ONE* 8: e76748.

Dulik, M.C., S.I. Zhadanov, L.P. Osipova, A. Askapuli, L. Gau, O. Gokcumen, S. Rubinstein, and T.G. Schurr. 2012. Mitochondrial DNA and Y chromosome variation provides evidence for a recent common ancestry between Native Americans and Indigenous Altaians. *American Journal of Human Genetics* 90: 229–246.

Gao, Zihou. 2000. The source, evolution and important impacts of Mongolic subgroups of the Yugurs. In *Studies of the Yugur ethnic group in China*, ed. Zhong Jinwen, 133–137. Minzu chubanshe: Beijing.

Ji, Yonghai. 2004. From contact to admixture-on the decline of the Manchu language (1). *Manchu Studies*. 1: 24–34.

Ji, Yonghai. 2005. From contact to admixture-on the decline of the Manchu language (2). *Manchu Studies* 1: 49–55.

Kharkova, V.N., K.V. Khaminaa, O.F. Medvedevaa, K.V. Simonovaa, E.R. Ereminab, and V.A. Stepanova. 2014. Gene Pool of Buryats: Clinal Variability and Territorial Subdivision Based on Data of Y-Chromosome Markers. *Russian Journal of Genetics* 50: 180–190.

Li, Keyu. 2008. *Collections of studies on the Tu people's history and languages*. Beijing: Minzu chubanshe.

Li, S. 2010. *Research on Oghuz and Uighur*. Beijing: Nationalities Publishing House.

Lin, Gan, and Gao Zihou. 1994. *History of the Old Uyghurs*. Huhhot: Neimenggu renmin chubanshe.

Liu, Yingsheng 2003 A brief review of the evolution of the Hui language -from Persian to Hui Chinese. *Studies of Chinese culture*. Winter tome, 143–153.

Malyarchuk, B., M. Derenko, G. Denisova, M. Wozniak, T. Grzybowski, I. Dambueva, and I. Zakharov. 2010. Phylogeography of the Y-chromosome haplogroup C in northern Eurasia. *Annals of Human Genetics* 74: 539–546.

Menhedalai and Huang Xing 1997. Analysis of the cognate distribution in the basic vocabulary of Mongolic and Turkish languages. *Minzu yuwen* [Non-Han languages] 1: 45–51.

Mi, Yizhi. 1981. Exploration of the origin and migration of the Salar. *Qinghai minzu xueyuan xuebao [Journal of the Institute of Qinghai Minorities]* 3: 59–66.

Qie, Pai. 2009. *Studies of peaceful cohabitation of multiple ethnicities and their trends of development in the Hexi Corridor*. Beijing: Minzu chubanshe.

Renfrew, C. 1987. *Archeology and Language*. Cambridge: Cambridge University Press.

Saliyanyu 2000. Yugurs in Jiuquan. In *Studies of the Yugur ethnic group in China*, ed. Zhong Jinwen, 592–594. Beijing: Minzu chubanshe.

Shi, H., H. Zhong, Y. Peng, Y.L. Dong, X.B. Qi, F. Zhang, L.F. Liu, S.J. Tan, R.Z. Ma, C.J. Xiao, R.S. Wells, L. Jin, and B. Su. 2008. Y chromosome evidence of earliest modern human settlement in East Asia and multiple origins of Tibetan and Japanese populations. *BMC Biology* 6: 45.

Shou, W.H., E.F. Qiao, C.Y. Wei, Y.L. Dong, S.J. Tan, H. Shi, W.R. Tang, and C.J. Xiao. 2010. Y-chromosome distributions among populations in Northwest China identify significant contribution from Central Asian pastoralists and lesser influence of western Eurasians. *Journal of Human Genetics* 55: 314–322.

Sun, Zhu, et al. 1990. *Dictionary of Mongolic languages*. Xining: Qinghai renmin chubanshe.

Wang, C.C., and H. Li. 2013. Inferring human history in East Asia from Y chromosomes. *Investig Genet* 4 (1): 11.

Wang, C.C., L.X. Wang, R. Shrestha, M. Zhang, X.Y. Huang, K. Hu, L. Jin, and H. Li. 2014. Genetic structure of Qiangic populations residing in the western Sichuan corridor. *PLoS ONE* 9 (8): e103772.

Wells, R.S., N. Yuldasheva, R. Ruzibakiev, P.A. Underhill, I. Evseeva, J. Blue-Smith, L. Jin, B. Su, R. Pitchappan, S. Shanmugalakshmi, K. Balakrishnan, M. Read, N.M. Pearson, T. Zerjal, M.T. Webster, I. Zholoshvili, E. Jamarjashvili, S. Gambarov, B. Nikbin, A. Dostiev, O. Aknazarov, P. Zalloua, I. Tsoy, M. Kitaev, M. Mirrakhimov, A. Chariev, and W.F. Bodmer. 2001. The Eurasian heartland: A continental perspective on Y-chromosome diversity. *Proceedings of the National Academy of Sciences of the United States of America* 98: 10244–10249.

Wen, B., H. Li, D. Lu, X. Song, F. Zhang, Y. He, F. Li, Y. Gao, X. Mao, L. Zhang, J. Qian, J. Tan, J. Jin, W. Huang, R. Deka, B. Su, R. Chakraborty, and L. Jin. 2004. Genetic evidence supports demic diffusion of Han culture. *Nature* 431: 302–305.

Wen, S.Q., X.D. Xie, and D. Xu. 2013. Contact and admixture-the relationship between Dongxiang population and their language viewed from Y chromosomes. *Yi Chuan* 35 (6): 761–770.

Xie, G.X., and X.P. Wang. 2009. *History of Gansu Kazakh*. Lanzhou: Gansu Cultural Publishing House.

Xu, Dan. 2014. *Tangwang hua yanjiu* [Studies of the Tangwang language] Beijing: Minzu chubanshe.

Yang, F. 2003. *Uighur literature and Uighur culture*. Beijing: Nationalities Publishing House.

Zerjal, T., Y. Xue, G. Bertorelle, R.S. Wells, W. Bao, S. Zhu, R. Qamar, Q. Ayub, A. Mohyuddin, S. Fu, P. Li, N. Yuldasheva, R. Ruzibakiev, J. Xu, Q. Shu, R. Du, H. Yang, M.E. Hurles, E. Robinson, T. Gerelsaikhan, B. Dashnyam, S.Q. Mehdi, and C. Tyler-Smith. 2003. The genetic legacy of the Mongols. *American Journal of Human Genetics* 72: 717–721.

Zhang, Z. 1991. *History of Gansu Yugur*. Lanzhou: Gansu Cultural Publishing House.

Zhaonasitu. 1981a. *Outline of the Tu language*. Beijing: Minzu chubanshe.

Zhaonasitu. 1981b. *Brief records of East Yugur language (in Chinese)*. Beijing: Nationalities Publishing House.

Zhong, H., H. Shi, X.B. Qi, Z.Y. Duan, P.P. Tan, L. Jin, B. Su, and R.Z. Ma. 2011. Extended Y chromosome investigation suggests postglacial migrations of modern humans into East Asia via the northern route. *Molecular Biology and Evolution* 28 (1): 717–727.

Zhong, H., H. Shi, X.B. Qi, C.J. Xiao, L. Jin, R.Z. Ma, and B. Su. 2010. Global distribution of Y-chromosome haplogroup C reveals the prehistoric migration routes of African exodus and early settlement in East Asia. *Journal of Human Genetics* 55: 428–435.

Zhou, Weizhou. 2004. The past and present of Northwest China's minority multiculture. *Xibei minzu luncong [Studies of Northwestern minorities]* 3: 1–45.

Relationship Between Altaic Speaking Populations and Their Languages Viewed from Y Chromosomes

Shaoqing Wen, Xiaodong Xie and Dan Xu

1 Introduction

Northwestern China includes the autonomous regions of Xinjiang and Ningxia and the provinces of Shaanxi, Gansu, and Qinghai. The Silk Road, a historical network of interlinking trade routes across the Afro-Eurasian landmass, passes through this region. A number of ethnic groups with different religious faiths, cultures and life customs inhabit in this region, and they have presumably experienced complicated histories: Han, Hui, Dongxiang, Bao'an, Tu, Eastern Yugur (Yugur, Enger), Western Yugur (Yugur, Saragh), Salar, Uygur, Tatar, Kirghiz, Kazakh, Ozbek, Tajik, Xibe, Mongolian, and Amdo Tibetan. From a linguistic point of view, Dongxiang, Bao'an, Tu and Eastern Yugur languages belong to the Mongolic group of the Altaic family, while Western Yugur, Uygur, Tatar, Kirghiz, Kazakh, Ozbek and Salar are part of the Turkic group in the same family; Xibe is classified within the Tungusic Group in the Altaic family (http://www.ethnologue.com/web.asp). However all linguists do not agree with the term "Altaic family". But as Norman points out, "A few European Turkologists remain skeptical about the Altaic theory, but among Mongolian and Tungusic specialists, the Altaic affinity is routinely accepted (Norman 1988)." It is clear that the term "Altaic family" is conventionally accepted by default because they cannot convince each other. The origin and classification of Altaic have long been controversial.

S. Wen (✉)
MOE Key Laboratory of Contemporary Anthropology, School of Life Sciences, Fudan University, Shanghai 200433, People's Republic of China
e-mail: wenshaoqing1982@gmail.com

X. Xie
The Institute of Genetics, Lanzhou University, Lanzhou 730000, People's Republic of China

S. Wen · D. Xu
Institut National des Langues et Civilisations Orientales (INALCO), CRLAO (CNRS), 63 Rue des Grands Moulins, Paris 75013, France

D. Xu and H. Li (eds.), *Languages and Genes in Northwestern China and Adjacent Regions*, DOI 10.1007/978-981-10-4169-3_5

The non–recombining portion of the Y chromosome, like the genetic markers of the mitochondrial genome, is a useful source of genetic data. The Y-linked loci in the NRYs are haploid, paternally inherited and devoid of recombination with the X-chromosome. Because of these particular characteristics, variation results in the accumulation of mutations over generations, which is called the paternal or male lineage. Population geneticists have extensively studied human male lineages to trace migrations and reconstruct human history (Wang and Li 2013; Wen et al. 2016). Furthermore, because it has been shown that the genetic diversity found in the Y-chromosome correlates better with linguistic classification than mitochondrial DNA does (Comas et al. 2008; Jean-Marie et al. 2009; Forster and Renfrew 2011), we have chosen Y-chromosome variation as the genetic marker in this study.

To explore the paternal genetic structure of Altaic-speaking populations in Northwestern China and to further investigate the relationship between the Altaic populations and their languages, we have performed detailed analyses of the extant local ethnic groups. In addition, we anticipate providing some valuable information for the reference of other disciplines.

2 Materials and Methods

2.1 *Population Samples*

The Y haplogroup data for Eastern Yugurs, Western Yugurs and Uygurs were derived from our previous studies (Zhou et al. 2007; Zhou et al. 2008), and those for the other Altaic-speaking populations were collected from reference journals (Xue et al. 2006; Shou et al. 2010). We used the following selection criteria: (1) sample size of no less than 30; and (2) populations with clearly stated ethnicity or geographic locations. Among the populations initially recruited with these criteria, several had more than one dataset from the same geographic or ethic group. The pairwise FST and associated P values of these datasets were first estimated from the haplogroup frequencies using the Arlequin 3.1 software (Excoffier et al. 2007). When the pairwise FST values were statistically insignificant ($P > 0.05$), the datasets were combined. Otherwise, each dataset was used independently.

The current study thus includes 964 individual samples from 20 populations. Populations were also grouped according to linguistic family into 8 Turkic, 5 Tungusic and 7 Mongolic populations (Table 1).

2.2 *Statistical Analyses*

The Y haplogroup of every individual was defined based on our previous studies and on the NRY haplogroup tree shown in the reference paper (Zhou et al. 2007;

Table 1 Source of data for 20 populations in this study

Population	Location	Language affiliation	References
Western Yugur	Gansu	Altaic, Turkic	Zhou et al. (2008)
Uygur-1	Urumqi, Xinjiang	Altaic, Turkic	Zhou et al. (2008), Xue et al. (2006)
Uygur-2	Yili, Xinjiang	Altaic, Turkic	Xue et al. (2006)
Tatar	Xinjiang	Altaic, Turkic	Shou et al. (2010)
Kirghiz	Xinjiang	Altaic, Turkic	Shou et al. (2010)
Kazakh	Xinjiang	Altaic, Turkic	Shou et al. (2010)
Ozbek	Xinjiang	Altaic, Turkic	Shou et al. (2010)
Salar	Qinghai	Altaic, Turkic	Shou et al. (2010)
Eastern Yugur	Gansu	Altaic, Mongolian	Zhou et al. (2008)
Tu	Qinghai	Altaic, Mongolian	Shou et al. (2010)
Bao'an	Gansu	Altaic, Mongolian	Shou et al. (2010)
Dongxiang	Gansu	Altaic, Mongolian	Shou et al. (2010)
Mongolian-1*	Inner Mongolian	Altaic, Mongolian	Xue et al. (2006), Shou et al. (2010)
Mongolian-2*	Outer Mongolian	Altaic, Mongolian	Xue et al. (2006)
Daur*	Heilongjiang	Altaic, Mongolian	Xue et al. (2006)
Xibe	Xinjiang	Altaic, Tungusic	Xue et al. (2006), Shou et al. (2010)
Ewenki*	Inner Mongolia	Altaic, Tungusic	Xue et al. (2006)
Hezhen*	Heilongjiang	Altaic, Tungusic	Xue et al. (2006)
Manchu*	Liaoning	Altaic, Tungusic	Xue et al. (2006)
Oroqen*	Heilongjiang	Altaic, Tungusic	Xue et al. (2006)

*Represent reference population

Zhou et al. 2008). The Arlequin 3.5.1.2 program was used to compute Fst distances and associated P values based on 10,000 permutations, and multidimensional scaling analysis (MDS) based on Fst matrix was carried out using the SPSS19.0 software package (SPSS, Chicago, IL) to show the genetic distances among the Altaic-speaking populations in Northwest China. The principal component (PC) analysis plots were also constructed in SPSS19.0 using data from the Y chromosome. Y haplogroup population dendrograms were constructed using the furthest neighbor method using SPSS19.0.

3 Results

3.1 Genetic Distance and MDS Analysis

We used Y-SNP haplogroup data to compute population genetic distances in the form of Fst values. The matrix of pairwise Fst values is shown in Fig. 1. The color

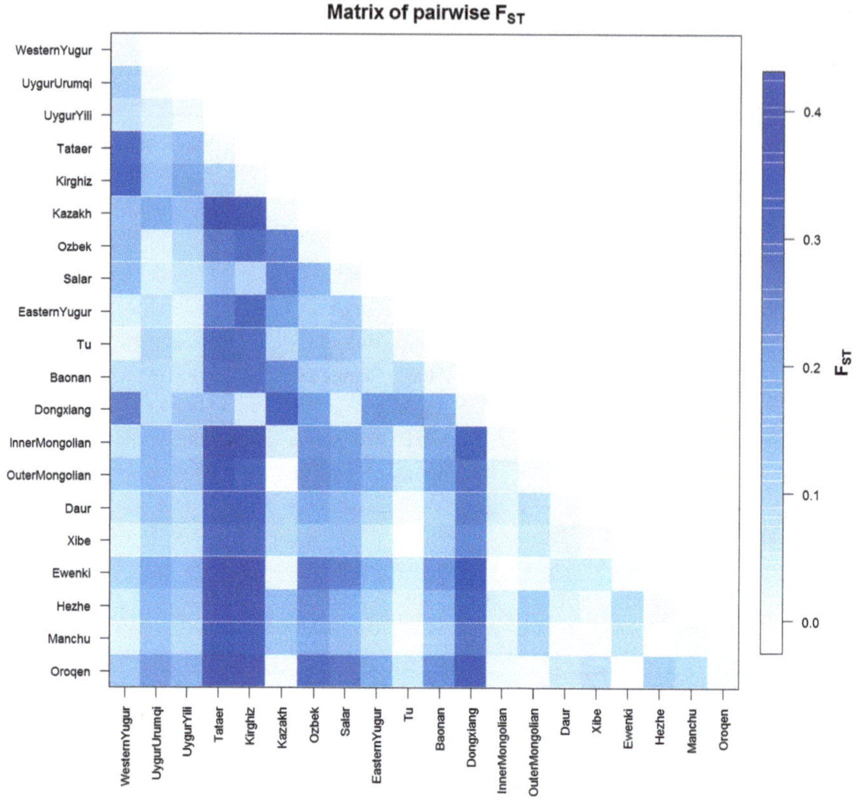

Fig. 1 Pairwise FSTs between populations. The color gradient indicates the relative degree of genetic distance from *white* (closer) to *blue* (farther)

gradient shows the relative level of genetic distance among the populations from white (closer) to blue (farther). In order to investigate the population genetic relationships, MDS analysis was performed on the basis of pairwise Fst values. Figure 2 shows the population distribution MDS plots. The Tungusic group and the Turkic group were placed close together, but the Mongolian group was not clearly separated from the Tungusic group or the Turkic group. The MDS plot indicates that the Tungusic and Turkic groups have large genetic distances from each other. The Mongolian group was close to the Tungusic group, and somewhat separate from Turkic Group. A good fit exists between the MDS plots and the source data.

3.2 Principal Component Analysis

Figure 3 shows the results of principal component (PC) analysis based on haplogroup frequencies for Y-SNP. PC analysis reveals that more than 67.2% of the

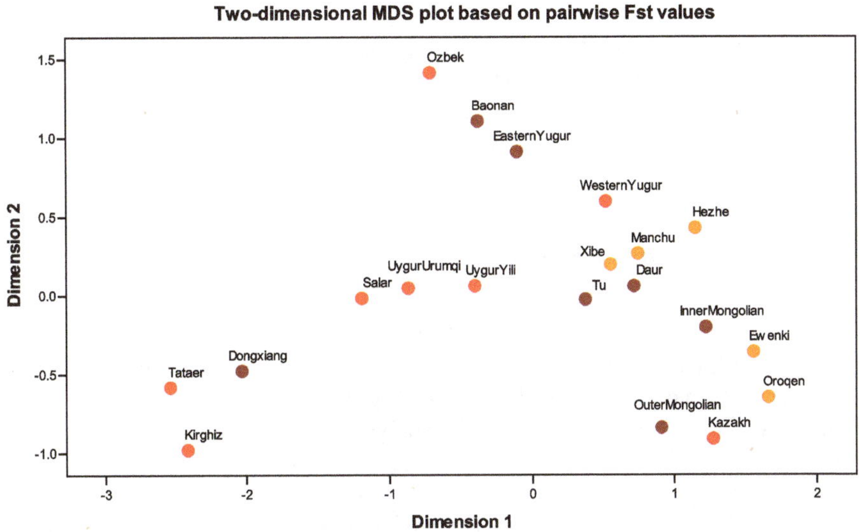

Fig. 2 Multidimensional scaling analysis of the Fst values. Altaic Family: *Orange circle* represents Tungusic Group; *Maroon circle* represents Mongolian Group; *Red circle* represents Turkic Group

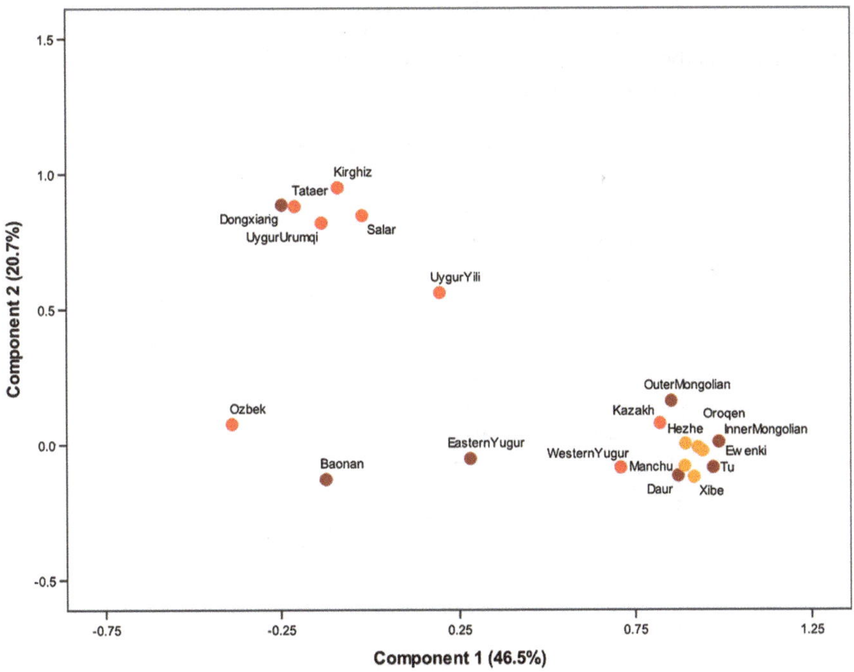

Fig. 3 Principal component (PC) analysis based on Y-SNP haplogroup frequencies. Altaic Family: *Orange circle* represents Tungusic group; *Maroon circle* represents Mongolian group; *Red circle* represents Turkic group

haplogroup variation is explained by the first two principal components. The population distribution in PC plots (Fig. 3) presents a similar genetic pattern to that in the MDS plots (Fig. 2). The Tungusic and Turkic groups are relatively well separated from each other. The Mongolian group, located between the Tungusic and Turkic groups in the plots, is slightly closer to the Tungusic Group.

3.3 Phylogenetic Analyses

In MDS analysis and PC analysis, the Tungusic and Turkic groups are relatively well separated, and the Mongolian group is slightly closer to the Tungusic Group. Dendrogram clustering can display the relationships among the populations in a different way from MDS analysis and PC analysis by giving an overall structure. In order to better understand the relationships, we constructed a phylogenetic tree (Fig. 4). Three clusters were created. The Mongolian-Tungusic group branch of Altaic, including the Tungusic group (Ewenki, Oroqen, Hezhen, Manchu and Xibe) and Mongolian group (Outer Mongolian, Inner Mongolian, Tu, Daur) fell into one cluster, with Kazakh close to them. The other two Mongolian group populations, Eastern Yugur and Bao'an, were clustered with the Turkic group. The last cluster contained the Dongxiang (belong to the Mongolian Group) and three Turkic-speaking populations. This result agrees with the results of the MDS analysis and PC analysis. The genetic structure is also generally consistent with linguistic classifications by linguists.

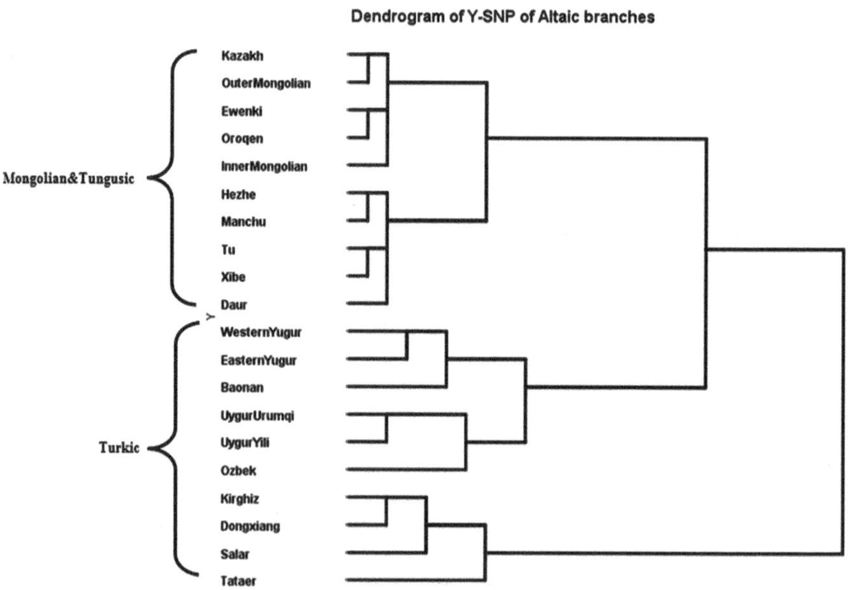

Fig. 4 Dendrogram of Y-SNP of Altaic branches

4 Conclusion

Genetic distance and MDS analysis indicate that certain differences exist between the Tungusic group and the Turkic group, and the Mongolian group is close to the Tungusic group (Figs. 1 and 2). The same results are also found in PC plots (Fig. 3). To further investigate the relationships among Altaic speaking populations and their languages, a dendrogram clustering has been constructed and its plot clearly shows the genetic relationships among the three clans of Altaic (Fig. 4). The significant genetic difference is possibly due to their different genetic origins. Genetic similarity between the two populations may result from various population history events. Because of the complexity of the Y chromosome marker system, it is highly unlikely that random genetic drift can lead to population similarity. So, if two populations originated from one common ancestral population, their genetic structures will be similar, and they are most reasonably classified into one group.

According to our analysis results, the genetic structure of Altaic speaking populations are generally consistent with linguistic classification, coinciding with other research using various scales (Piazza et al. 1995; Karafet et al. 2001; Tishkoff et al. 2009; Friedlaender et al. 2008; Wang et al. 2007). But there are some mismatches between paternal genetic lineage and language classification: for example, the Dongxiang people are much closer to the Turkic ethnic groups than to the other Mongolian groups (Wen et al. 2013). This exception in the correlation between genes and languages might be well explained by the elite-dominance model. In this case, a limited group of individuals have taken over the political, religious or social rule of a general population, imposing a new language. As a consequence, a linguistic replacement can take place without a genetic replacement of the population. This process is only possible in very structured populations with a social hierarchy, where the replacement of a small amount of leading individuals might affect the general population (Comas et al. 2008; Renfrew 1987; CavalliSforza 1997).

On the whole, the paternal lineages that have been observed in the Altaic ethnic groups of Northern China reveal two interesting facts: (i) the Tungusic ethnic groups and the Turkic ethnic groups display large genetic distances from each other; the Mongolian Group, located between the Tungusic Group and the Turkic Group in the MDS and PC plots, is comparatively close to the Tungusic Group and, (ii) the relationship between paternal genetic lineage and language classification among the Altaic-speaking populations of Northwest China is roughly parallel. Further studies considering more loci and Y-STR markers will help to further confirm the genetic relationships between these various Altaic groups, and complementary autosomal and mtDNA must also be performed in the future.

References

Cavalli-Sforza, L.L. 1997. Genes, peoples, and languages. *Proceedings of the National Academy of Sciences of the United States of America* 94 (15): 7719–7724.

Comas, D., et al. 2008. *Human Genetics and Languages*. Chichester: John Wiley & Sons.

Excoffier, L., et al. 2007. Arlequin (version 3.0): An integrated software package for population genetics data analysis. *Evolutionary Bioinformatics Online* 23 (1): 47–50.

Forster, P., and C. Renfrew. 2011. Mother Tongue and Y Chromosomes. *Science* 333 (6048): 1390–1391.

Friedlaender, J.S., et al. 2008. The genetic structure of Pacific Islanders. *PLoS Genetics* 4 (1): e19.

Jean-Marie, H., et al. 2009. *Becoming Eloquent: Advances in the emergence of language, human cognition, and modern cultures*. Amsterdam: John Benjamins Publishing Company.

Karafet, T., et al. 2001. Paternal population history of East Asia: Sources, patterns, and microevolutionary processes. *American Journal of Human Genetics* 69 (3): 615–628.

Norman, J. 1988. *Chinese*. Cambridge: Cambridge University Press.

Piazza, A., et al. 1995. Genetics and the origin of European languages. *Proceedings of the National Academy of Sciences of the United States of America* 92 (13): 5836–5840.

Renfrew, C. 1987. *Archeology and Language*. Cambridge: Cambridge Univ. Press.

Shou, W.H., et al. 2010. Y-chromosome distributions among populations in Northwest China identify significant contribution from Central Asian pastoralists and lesser influence of western Eurasians. *Journal of Human Genetics* 55 (5): 314–322.

Tishkoff, S.A., et al. 2009. The genetic structure and history of Africans and African Americans. *Science* 324 (5930): 1035–1044.

Wang, C.C., and H. Li. 2013. Inferring human history in East Asia from Y chromosomes. *Investigative Genetics* 4 (1): 11.

Wang, S., et al. 2007. Genetic variation and population structure in native Americans. *PLoS Genetics* 3 (11): e185.

Wen, S.Q., et al. 2013. Contact and admixture—the relationship between Dongxiang population and their language viewed from Y chromosomes. *Yi Chuan* 35 (6): 761–770.

Wen, S.Q., et al. 2016. Y-chromosome based genetic pattern in East Asia affected by Neolithic transition. Quaternary International (in press).

Xue, Y.L., et al. 2006. Male demography in East Asia: A north-south contrast in human population expansion times. *Genetics* 172 (4): 2431–2439.

Zhou, R., et al. 2007. Testing the hypothesis of an ancient Roman soldier origin of the Liqian people in northwest China: A Y-chromosome perspective. *Journal of Human Genetics* 52 (7): 584–591.

Zhou, R., et al. 2008. Origin and evolution of two Yugur sub-clans in Northwest China: A case study in paternal genetic landscape. *Annals of Human Biology* 35 (2):198–211.

Formation of a “Mixed Language” in Northwest China—the Case of Tangwang

Dan Xu and Shaoqing Wen

Abbreviations

1SG	1st personal pronoun singular
1PL	1st personal pronoun plural
2 SG	2nd personal pronoun singular
2 PL	2nd personal pronoun plural
3 SG	3rd personal pronoun singular
3 PL	3rd personal pronoun plural
ACC	Accusative
ABL	Ablative
CAUS	Causative
CL	Classifier
COM	Comitative
COMP	Comparative
CONV	Converb
DAT	Dative
INST	Instrumental
INTER	Interrogative particle
MOD-PART	Modal particle
PL	Plural
POSS	Possessive

D. Xu (✉) · S. Wen
Institut National des Langues et Civilisations Orientales (INALCO),
63 Rue des Grands Moulins, Paris 75013, France
e-mail: xusongdan@gmail.com

D. Xu
CRLAO (CNRS), Paris, France

S. Wen
MOE Key Laboratory of Contemporary Anthropology, School of Life Sciences,
Fudan University, Shanghai 200433, People’s Republic of China

D. Xu and H. Li (eds.), *Languages and Genes in Northwestern China and Adjacent Regions*, DOI 10.1007/978-981-10-4169-3_6

POST	Postposition
PRF	Perfect
REFL	Reflexive
RES	Resultative
TERM	Terminative

1 Introduction

Gansu Province borders Qinghai to the southwest and Xinjiang to the west; it is crossed by an anthropological and linguistic corridor where several ethnicities and languages are found. Known as the Hexi [west of the Yellow River] Corridor, it partially coincides with the famous Silk Road. At least nine ethnic groups are found in this corridor: Han (Chinese), Hui (Muslim), Dongxiang (Santa), Bao'an, Monguor (Tu), Eastern Yugur, Western Yugur, Salar, and Amdo Tibetan. These peoples speak languages belonging to two large language families: Chinese and Amdo Tibetan belong to the Sino-Tibetan family, and the Mongolic and Turkic languages belong to the Altaic family (the term "Altaic family" is taken in its traditional reading even though the debate on it continues).

Tangwang is located inside the autonomous district of Dongxiang (Santa) which belongs to Linxia Hui Autonomous Prefecture in the province of Gansu, China. Its longitude is 103°32', and its latitude is 35°47'. Its geographic conditions are suitable for human habitation: it is a relatively flat region along the downstream section of the Tao River, situated between mountains. The altitude is high, ranging from more than 1000 to 1700 m. Tangwang has a total area of 46 km^2, and is 8 km from east to west and 10 km from north to south (Figs. 1, 2).

The Tangwang language was first described in an article by Chen (1985, Ibramhim) in the journal *Minzu Yuwen* [Non-Han languages]. Why has this language generated great interest in the linguistic community? In China, it has been described as a "mixed language" (Sun et al. [eds.] 2007) based on the *Minzu Yuwen* article. In the West, this language was almost unknown because not all linguists read articles in Chinese. The Tangwang language should actually be divided into two varieties, one spoken by converts to Islam (called Hui in Tangwang), and the other by non-Muslims, the remaining Han people. Actually, the Tangwang language often refers to that spoken by Hui people.[1] It shares the characteristics of other languages in this region, having predominantly Chinese vocabulary with some words borrowed from Arabic and Mongolian. The word order is predominantly SOV (subject-object-verb), an order which is common to all Altaic languages, while SVO is also accepted in some cases (recall that the word order in Chinese is SVO). The languages in this region all borrowed their case system from Mongolic languages (or dialects), while Chinese is a morphologically poor

[1]However we will succinctly present what has happened among Han people if necessary.

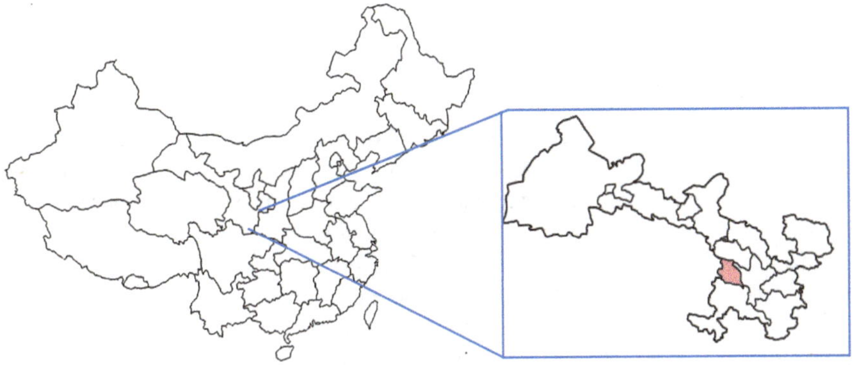

Fig. 1 Linxia Hui autonomous prefecture in Gansu, China

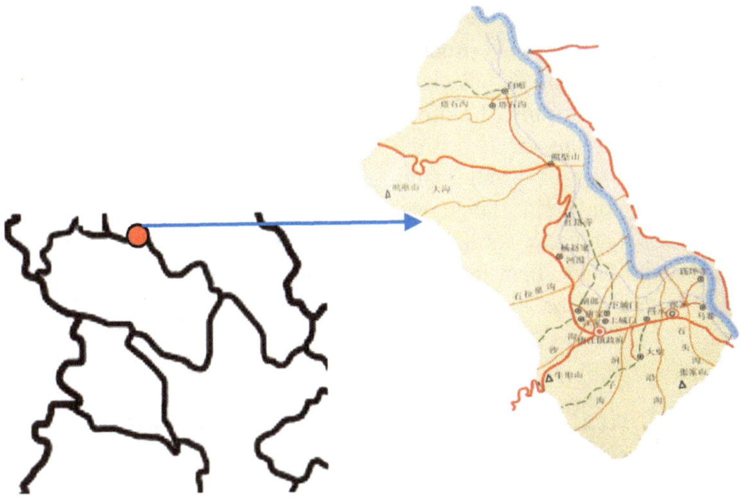

Fig. 2 Map of Tangwang. The map of Tangwang is drawn from the *Zhangjiacun zhi* [Annals of the Zhang family] (2004)

language with no case system. The languages in this region are in the process of losing their tones, and the degree of loss varies from region to region, while Standard Chinese has four tones. The Dongxiang (Santa) language has surrounded the Tangwang people for some hundreds of years, and Dongxiang language influence is inevitable.

Within the historical context of East-West exchanges, present-day populations in this area show a high level of both linguistic and genetic diversity, indicating that their languages and genetic makeup may be associated with complex processes of linguistic contact and population admixture. Our article deals with the Tangwang language and the formation of the Tangwang people. In presenting Xu’s field work and research (Xu 2014) along with Wen Shaoqing's genetic analysis of the main families in Tangwang, we are reporting on the first results of our studies of this language and people.

According to our preliminary research, a solely linguistic approach is insufficient; an interdisciplinary approach is required. We have attempted to combine a linguistic approach with a biological one, to better understand the coevolution of language and genes. The Tangwang language has been investigated in our previous linguistic studies (Xu 2014), and there are relatively clear historical records of the origins of the Tangwang people; thus the Tangwang people and their language are an ideal model for studying language contact and formation of a new population.

In this study, we first collected 151 male samples from 5 family clans (with surnames Tang, Wang, Zhang, Yang and Zhao) in the town of Tangwang in Linxia Hui Autonomous Prefecture, Gansu Province, to trace the origin and demographic history of the Tangwang people, and then investigated 96 linguistic features of the Tangwang language and other reference languages in China.

Our results show that: (1) the Tangwang language is not yet a mixed language, even though its Chinese syntax structure shows some influence from the Dongxiang (Santa) language, (2) Almost all the clans have dominant paternal lineages associated with different origins; the times to most recent common ancestor of the 5 clans coincide with the local records of historical settlement; (3) based on 96 linguistic features, the Tangwang language tends to cluster with Sinitic languages rather than with non-Sinitic languages. Overall, we can employ the principle of coevolution of language, Y chromosome and clan to reconstruct the formation of a mixed population and their languages, and to further study the relationships between language contact and population admixture.

2 The Historical and Ethnic Context of Tangwang

To better understand the people of Tangwang, it is necessary to briefly present the Dongxiang people, whose language exerts a strong influence on the Tangwang language. In both the linguistic and genetic domain, Dongxiang merits attention. We (Xu et al. 2013) have shown that the Persian, Arabic and Turkic lexical elements in the Dongxiang (Santa) language are not loanwords, but are rather relics from the substratum language spoken by their forefathers, who were related to the people of Central Asia. Historical and cultural evidence also tells us that some of the Dongxiang people's ancestors came from Central Asia, and some from Western Asia; they may have come from different branches and ethnic origins. The Dongxiang language is the result of contact between different languages and cultures. The biological tests and analyses converge with linguistic and historical data.

In Tangwang, the two major families are Tang and Wang. Some minor family names are Zhang, Yang and Zhao. Historical documents such as Tang Hanqing's *Memoirs*, (manuscript) 1987, and the chronicles of the Zhang Family (see Zhangjiacun zhi 2004), indicate that the Yang and Zhao families were earlier

Chart 1 Population growth

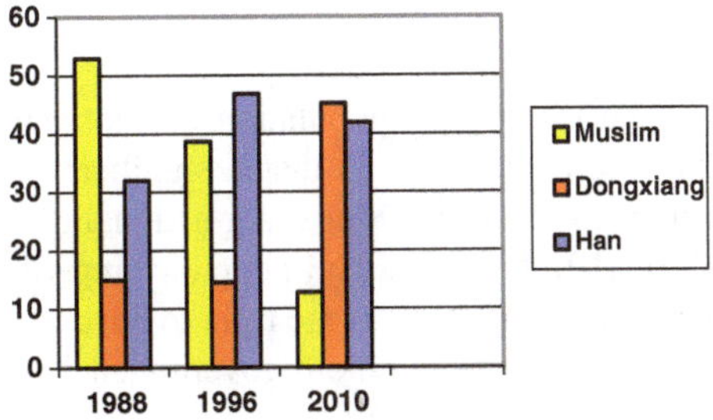

Chart 2 Comparison of Muslim and Han populations

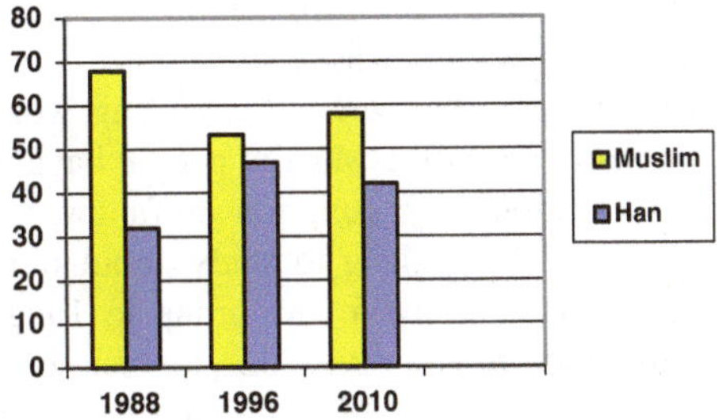

inhabitants of Tangwang. The Tang clan settled in this region around late Yuan dynasty (1206–1368) when some members of the Tang family converted to Islam. Today those who have not adopted Islam have stayed in Xiachuan (which is also called Sanhe), while those who did convert have gathered in Shangchuan, which is considered the center of Tangwang (where the township government is located). The Wang clan arrived after the Tang family, no later than in early Ming dynasty (1368–1644). The members of the Wang family helped the Tang during the repression of Muslims by the Qing government in 1781, and since that event, the two families have formed an alliance and have led a friendly coexistence into the present day.

The distribution of Muslim and Han people is important to understanding the mentalities of the Tangwang people.[2] In 2010, the Dongxiang population made up 45.2% of the population, the Hui people (Muslim) 12.8%, Han 41.92%, and some people belonging to peripheral ethnicities 0.046%. The Dongxiang and Hui are both Muslim, and together they account for 58% of the total. Xu's field work (2014) reveals that the proportion of Han (Chinese) to Muslim has undergone some

[2]Tang Zhi' statistics (2011) based on those of the Office of the Tangwang Government in 2011 are slightly different from those collected by Xu in 2010 from the Family Records Department of the Tangwang Public Security Bureau. The proportion is almost the same, but the total number is smaller; for example, the population in Tangwang was 14107 according to the Office of the Tangwang Government, while it was 15093 according to the Family Records Department of the Tangwang Public Security Bureau. Here we take the data provided by Xu in 2010.

changes over the past three decades. Observe the following charts drawn from Xu (2014) (Charts 1, 2).

The Dongxiang population did not actually increase so quickly. The most reasonable explanation is that a significant number of Hui Muslims declared themselves to be of the Dongxiang nationality. Tang Zhi (a native of Tangwang) reveals (2011:19) that some Hui people change their nationality to Dongxiang in order to get advantages such as the right to have more children and other benefits awarded to minorities by the Chinese government.[3] Still according to him, people declare their nationality as they want; it sometimes happens that brothers or sisters in the same family have different ethnic identities, one Hui and the other Dongxiang. This means that the Dongxiang people of Tangwang did not necessarily originate from Dongxiang people, whose ancestors, as we have mentioned, came from Central and Western Asia. Numerous Dongxiang women have settled in Tangwang through intermarriage. Some Muslim people have changed their nationality to Dongxiang. This situation is so common in Tangwang that we have to use the term Muslim rather than Dongxiang to study populations located in Tangwang. Muslim populations have formed a core group in Tangwang. Han people and Muslims are in harmonious relationships due to their common history. However intermarriages only occur between Muslims, never with Han people, for religious reasons. It is easy to imagine that since many Muslim people in Tangwang have changed their nationality to Dongxiang, most Muslim people were non-Muslim in the past. Local elders unanimously recognize that their forefathers were Han but not Muslim. This specific historical factor prevents ethnic or religious conflicts among the people of Tangwang.

There are various legends about the origin of the Tang family. In Tang (1987) *Memoirs*, the common ancestor of the Tang family was a retired military official of the Mongolian Army who was the first Tang immigrant in this region, where the Yang and Zhao families were older inhabitants. Still according to Tang Hanqing, the Yang, Zhao and Zhang families were Han. Our genetic analysis reveals that their origins are different from what people have believed, but at least the manuscript of Tang Hanqing suggests that these populations were already Sinicized. As for the Mongolian military official, two versions of the story of his marriage circulate among the Tang family: one is that he married a woman named Zhao, and the other is that he took a Mongolian woman as his wife. These two legends do not exclude the possibility that his first wife was named Zhao while his second wife (the order may be different) indeed was a Mongolian woman. The oral legends have to be taken seriously, since they often provide us traces of their ancestors' origins. One thing is particularly amazing: almost all people of the Tang family told us that this Mongolian Army official had a Han origin and came from Sichuan, but no one doubts that his origin is Mongolian. See analysis about their genes in Sect. 4.

[3]China's one-child policy began in the 1980's, but it does not apply to minorities.

3 Linguistic Situation in Tangwang

The Tangwang language, a language island in Dongxiang County, should be classified within Hezhou (or Linxia) dialect. The geographical range of Hezhou dialect includes several districts and cities west of the Tao River in Gansu: Linxia district and Linxia city, Hezheng, Guanghe, Yongjing, and some locations in Qinghai such as Ledu, Minhe, Xunhua and Tongren. The Tangwang language is isolated from other Chinese dialects (separated from Chinese dialects by the Tao River to the east and surrounded by the Dongxiang (Santa) language. Language contact in Tangwang has been and still is intensive, and the languages in contact belong to two unrelated language families: Chinese, which is in the Sino-Tibetan family, and Dongxiang of the Altaic family. Although the Chinese language is in a dominant position, it has begun to change and to absorb some alien elements. The Tangwang language, which apparently originated from Mandarin, clearly shows parallel and regular evolution in phonology with other Chinese dialects (see Xu 2015a). It is becoming a language with morphological case, while contemporary Chinese languages do not use case at all (though in Old Chinese, traces of case use might exist). What happened in this area is quite remarkable. Some other languages show scenarios similar to Tangwang: borrowing is not limited to words and word orders, but also includes morphology and even parts of the phonological system. At a syntactic level, these languages have changed from SVO word order to SOV order. Morphologically, these languages have begun to develop a case marking system, and mark plurality regardless of a noun's human feature. These new morphological and syntactic means are clearly different from other Sinitic languages. As for the phonological system, which is in general the most resistant to change, some languages in this region have begun the process of simplification of tones, or have even lost the tone system, while tones are phonemic in Chinese. Li 1983, Chen 1985, Dwyer 1992; Janhunen 2004, Janhunen et al. 2008, Xu 2011, among others reveal that in Northwest China, the Chinese language has undergone important changes due to language contact. The influence is not a one-way process; both the Chinese language and non-Han languages are undergoing profound changes in this region.

The Tangwang phonological system contains eight basic vowels: i,y,u,e,ə,ɛ,ɔ,a and 23 consonants: p, ph, t, th, k, kh, m, n (ɳ), f, v (ʋ), s, ʂ, ʐ, ɕ, x (χ), ts, tsh, tʂ, tʂh, tɕ, tɕh, l, j (ʑ). The symbols in parentheses are allophones and are not counted as phonemes. More concretely, v and ʋ, n and ɳ, j and ʑ, and x and χ are allophones. In these four pairs, the first symbol is the basic phoneme and the second is its allophone. ʋ and χ are free allophones with v and x, while ɳ and ʑ are phonetically conditioned ones (see details in Xu 2014). Several phonetic characteristics are salient. (1) The friction is stronger than that in Standard Mandarin. When a bilabial 'p' precedes a close front vowel, 'p' almost becomes 'ps'. The alveolars 't, th' in Standard Mandarin are systematically converted into the affricates 'tɕ, tɕh' when they are followed by close front vowels. This phonetic change is also attested in Linxia (cf the reference on Linxia dialect) and Urumqi dialects (Liu Lili 1989), and in the Donggan language (Lin Tao 2009). When 't' or 'th' precedes other vowels (non-front, non-close vowels), it remains 't' or 'th' in Tangwang. The aspirated plosives 'ph' and 'th' behave differently depending on the following vowel. This is also attested in other dialects in Gansu. (2) The Mandarin diphtongs ai, ao, ei become ɛ, e, ɔ in Tangwang. This phenomenon is widely attested in Chinese dialects in Gansu and Qinghai provinces (see Ma 1984 for Hezhou dialect, Zhang 2006 for Qinghai dialects among others). (3) Nasals do not occur at the end of a word; nasalization takes place in the preceding vowel. (4) Under influence from the Dongxiang language, tone is almost lost in young Muslim speakers when reading *single words*, while in the Han population the tone system is simplified (see Chen 1999, Xu 2014 among others). At the morphological and syntactic levels, the Tangwang language possesses case markers (accusative/dative, ablative, instrumental/comitative). Some morphological suffixes which typically belong to Mongolic languages are attested in Tangwang among the Muslim population and have not yet been adopted by Han settlers, i.e. people in Tangwang who have not converted to Islam. The syntax is similar to Mongolic languages with OV order and converbs used to link two sentences. The vocabulary is mainly Chinese scattered with a few words from Arabic, Persian and Turkic sources, specially used in Muslim religious contexts. Apparently these words have entered through the Dongxiang language.

Based on our own field research, we believe that the language has not yet completed the mixing process, although some grammatical means such as case markers, and some suffixes which are alien to Chinese languages and dialects, are well-attested in the Tangwang language. The vocabulary remains Chinese with some co-existing syntactic doublets (Chinese and non-Chinese).

Here we present some examples, first illustrating different word orders, then showing case marking. For a full description of the Tangwang language, readers are invited to consult the monograph on the Tangwang language by Xu (2014).

-Word order

The most frequent word order is O (object) + V (verb), just as in other Sinitic languages in this region (Linxia, Xining among others). VO order is also attested, but mainly in fixed expressions. Now let us observe some OV sentences:

(1) 羊们哈赶着进来给。

jɑ̃ mu xa kɛ̃ tʂə tɕĩlɛ kɪ
sheep PL ACC pursue CONV enter CAUS
'Herd these sheep into the pen.'

(2) 阿訇两个鸡哈宰哈了。

axũ liɑ̃ ke tɕi xa tsɛ xa liɔ
imam two CL chicken ACC kill RES PRF
'The imam has killed two chickens.'

(3) 我你哈花哈给一个。

və ȵa xa xua xa kha ʑi ke
1SG 2SG + DAT DAT flower ACC give one CL
'I gave you one flower.'

In the above examples, the word order is OV. The accusative marker [xa] marks the preverbal object. It is clear that the object can be either definite or indefinite. The plural marker [mu], equivalent to [mən] in Standard Mandarin, can mark a noun with the inanimate feature. This kind of plural marking is impossible in Mandarin except in fairy tales. In a double object construction such as in (3), both objects can be marked. In the corpus collected by Xu (2014), the indirect object is marked in a double object construction, while the direct object can dispense with the marking. This phenomenon is also found in Qinghai dialect (see Ren 2004).

-Case marking

Case marking is one of the most striking characteristics of the Tangwang language when compared to Mandarin. The case markers include ones which are attested in almost all Mongolic language groups. In the Tangwang language, the nominative marker takes the null form (just as in other Mongolic languages) while the accusative and dative markers take the same phonetic form [xa] which is also a homophone with an aspectual particle and the topic marker. This is quite different from Mongolic languages in which dative and locative markers share the same morpheme. The Tangwang language also has an ablative marker [ɕiɛ], which is also used in comparative sentences, and [la] which is employed as an instrumental marker after a noun with the [-Animate] feature, or as a comitative marker when used after a noun with the [+ A] feature. We continue with some examples:

(4) 羊哈狼吃上了。

jɑ̃ xa lɑ̃ tʂhʅ-ɑ̃ liɔ
sheep ACC wolf eat RES PRF
'The sheep has been eaten by the wolf.'

(5) 小王小李哈打哈了。

ɕiɔ vɑ̃ ɕiɔ li xa ta xa liɔ
Xiao Wang Xiao Li ACC beat RES PRF
'Xiao Wang has beaten Xiao Li.'

In (4), the nominative [lɑ̃] 'wolf' is unmarked while the object [jɑ̃] 'sheep' must be marked by [xa]. The same analysis is applied to (5) in which two nouns with the [+ A] feature require a marker to distinguish the agent from the patient. Notice that case marking affects the pronunciation of the 1st and 2nd person pronouns:

(6) 你我看来了?

ȵi va kɛ̃ lɛ liɔ
2SG 1SG + ACC see come PRF
'Did you come to see me?'

(7) 我你说。

və ŋ̊a ʂuə
1SG 2SG + DAT say
'I speak to you.'

When the first person pronoun is used in subject position, it is pronounced [və], while when it is used in object position (in Tangwang the object is preverbal), it becomes [va]. The second person is ŋ̊i in subject position and ŋ̊a in object position, respectively. Now look at additional case marking such as ablative/comparative and instrumental/comitative.

(8) 我家里些来了。

və tɕia li ɕiɛ lɛ liɔ
1SG home POST ABL come PRF
'I have come from my home.'

(9) 马驴些快。

ma ly ɕiɛ khuɛ
horse donkey COMP fast
'The horse runs faster than the donkey.'

(10) 那蒙古话拉讲。

nə mə̃ku xua la tɕiɑ̃
3SG Mongol speech INST speak
'He speaks Mongolian.'

(11) 那ake拉走了?

nə ake la tsəu liɔ
3SG who COM go INTER
'With whom did he go?'

According to our research, the Tangwang language developed among Han people and some Sinicized Mongolian people (in the Tang family), but not from Dongxiang (Santa) people's language. Dongxiang people learn the Chinese language as a target language. Some scholars have confused the Dongxiang population with those in Tangwang who have declared their own identity as Dongxiang. Our studies clearly show that the Tangwang people and the Dongxiang population do not share the same Y-chromosome haplogroups (see next section).

According to our previous studies (Xu et al. 2013), genetic distance calculations show that of 93 populations on the Eurasian continent, the ethnic groups with the closest affinity to the Dongxiang are the Tajik (Khojant), Tajike (Xinjiang), Salar, Ishkashimi, Kirghiz (Xinjiang), and Bartangi. In other words, Dongxiang's ancestors mainly came from Central Asia (some from West Asia) while in Tangwang, neither from the two most important families Tang and Wang, nor from other less significant clans, the Central Asia contribution is substantial (0.6% in the

Tang family, 2.6% in the Zhang family). Judging by their Y-chromosomes, some Dongxiang people in Tangwang are among those who have recently declared themselves to be Dongxiang.

4 Genetic Origins of the People of Tangwang

Materials and Methods A clan-based genetic investigation had been carried out in the town of Tangwang in Linxia Hui Autonomous Prefecture, Gansu Province. 151 saliva samples of Tangwang residents, including 30 males with the surname Yang, 30 males with the surname Zhao, 31 males with the surname Zhang, 30 males with the surname Tang and 30 males with the surname Wang, were collected and analyzed in this study, with informed consent. Our study was approved by the Ethnic Committee of the School of Life Sciences, Fudan University.

Y chromosome haplogroup profile As shown in Fig. 3, except for the Zhao clan, each clan has its own dominant paternal lineage: D3a-P47 (33.33%) in the surname Yang, H-M69 (60%) in the surname Zhang, C3*-ST (53.33%) in the surname Tang and O3a1c-002611(73.33%) in the surname Wang. Haplogroup D is comprised of subclades D1-M15 and D3-P99 in continental East Asia, and is especially frequent in Tibetan Haplogroup D1-M15 (Shi, H. et al. 2008), which is seen as a widely distributed Paleolithic genetic legacy among most Tibeto-Burman, Tai-Kadai, and Hmong-Mien populations (Shi et al. 2008, Qi 2013). Haplogroup D is only found once in the Wang clan, while D3a-P47, exclusively distributed in Tibeto-Burman populations (Shi et al. 2008,) is prevalent in the Yang (33.33%), Zhao (25.81%), Zhang (13.33%) and Tang (10%) clans. As the Yang and Zhao clans were the

Fig. 3 Sample collections in Tangwang

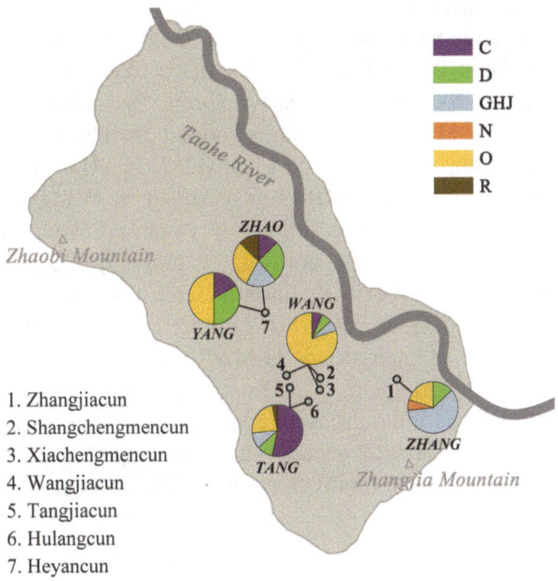

earliest settlers in the town of Tangwang according to historical records, this distribution of frequencies among the different clans reflects the early influence of Tibeto-Burman populations.

Haplogroup C may represent one of the initial groups of migrants to East Eurasia and Australia. Haplogroup C3-M217 is the most widespread subclade, and reaches the highest frequencies among Altaic-speaking populations, e.g. Mongol, Manchu, and Kazakh (Zhong et al. 2010). However, it is worthwhile to note that Haplogroup C3 comprises two clades: one is the northern clade, defined by SNP F1396, which is frequently found in Mongol and Manchu populations; the other is the southern clade, defined by SNP F2613, which is found mainly in Han Chinese (Yan et al. 2014). In this study, four F2613-derived individuals were found in the Zhao clan, suggesting a recent gene flow or migration from Han Chinese populations; other C3 samples (16.67% in the Yang clan, 53.33% in the Tang clan and 3.33% in the Wang clan) belong to downstream haplogroups of the northern clade, especially star-cluster (C3*xC3c), which is abundant in the steppe ethnicities and is even hypothesized to consist of Genghis Khan's descendants (Zerjal et al. 2003), indicating a substantial genetic contribution from Mongolian-speaking populations. This result coincides with the written records, as mentioned above, which say that the common ancestor of the Tang clan was a retired general in the late Yuan dynasty.

Haplogroup O-M175 and its brother haplogroup N-M231 are the dominant Y chromosome macrohaplogroups in Han Chinese. The former covers a quarter of the males in the world today. O3a1c-02611, O3a2c1-M134, and O3a2c1a-M117 are three main subclades of O3-M122 (a downstream marker of O-M175), each accounting for 12–17% of the Han Chinese population (Wang and Li 2013). Significantly, they exhibit various frequencies in the five clans. Haplogroup O3a1c-002611 reaches its highest frequency (73.33%) in the Wang clan, but is nearly absent in the other four clans, which means that the ancestors of the Wang clan might have been recent Han immigrants. Haplogroup O3a2c1*-M134 accounts for about 20% of the samples in the Yang clan and 12.9% of the Zhao clan, respectively, but is nearly absent in other clans. Similarly, Haplogroup O3a2c1a-M117 only exhibits modest frequencies (6.67%) in the Yang clan. So, haplogroup O3a2c1*-M134 and O3a2c1a-M117 are prevalent in Yang clan, while haplogroup O3a1c-002611 is frequent in Wang clan. This difference might be caused by the various origins of Yang and Wang clans, as modern Sino-Tibetan populations share the dominant haplogroup O3a2c1*-M134 and O3a2c1a-M117 (Wang et al. 2014) while Eastern Han Chinese display relatively high frequencies of haplogroup O3a1c-002611(Wang 2013). The rest of the Y chromosomes were identified as haplogroups G-M201, H-M69, J-P209, and R-M207, and we define these haplogroups as West Eurasian related haplogroups because they occur preferentially in West Eurasian populations (Wang and Li 2013). It is noteworthy that haplogroup H-M69 occurs with high frequency only in the Zhang clan. The haplotypes of H-M69 individuals in the Zhang clan are more similar to samples from the surrounding Muslim populations (unpublished data), such as Hui, Dongxiang and Bao’an, who were Persian and Arab immigrants from Central Asia during Yuan Dynasty (approximately 700 years ago).

5 Status of the Tangwang Language with Respect to Other Languages in China

As has been indicated in the previous sections, the Tangwang language is a Chinese variety influenced by the Dongxiang language, but it is not the result of imperfect acquisition of the Mandarin language by Dongxiang people. The Tangwang language is classified as a “mixed language” in *Languages in China* (Sun et al. [eds.] 2007). Linguists do not yet possess a universally adopted method to define “mixed language”. Thomason et al.(1988) have established a borrowing scale including five degrees or categories; but as these authors indicate: “The boundaries between any two borrowing categories on our scale are of course fuzzy” (p. 77). In our field investigations, the real linguistic data often presents much more intermediate phases. In their highest category of borrowing scale, i.e. degree five, they describe the following:

> 5) Very strong cultural pressure: heavy structural borrowing; structure:
> Major structural features that cause significant typological disruption: …loss of phonemic contrasts; change in word structure rules (e.g. adding prefixes in a language that was exclusively suffixing… (p76).

In the Tangwang language, some phenomena correspond to these criteria but some do not. As for typological change in *heavy structural borrowing*, the Tangwang language has changed from VO word order to OV word order. In our experience, this is not very significant, since word order is one of the most easily changed features in language contact. As we have mentioned in Sect. 2, the Tangwang language has begun to lose tone in single words, which is Thomason and Kaufman’s *loss of phonemic contrasts*. It is well known that contemporary Chinese does not appeal to morphology as do European languages. However the Tangwang language, which is spoken by people who have converted to Islam,[4] has begun to use morphological suffixes—more precisely, grammatical suffixes. This is completely alien to Sinitic languages, even in the linguistic area around the border between Gansu and Qinghai. Here are a few examples:

(12) 我家里nə去咧。

və tɕa li nə tɕhi lɛ
1SG home POST REFL go MOD-PART
‘I’m going home’

[4]Those who have not converted to Islam do not completely accept these suffixes.

Chart 3 Reflexive and possessive suffixes

	Tangwang	Dongxiang (Santa)
Reflexive	-nə	-nə
	Cooccurrence with case markers	*Ibid* except accusative
3SG POSS	-ɳ̩i	-ni
	Only 3SG	mini (1SG) matanni (incl), (1PL) bitʑiənni (excl),(1PL) tʂɯni (2SG), tani (2PL) ni (3SG/PL)

(13) 书ɳ̩i破哈寨

ʂu ɳ̩i pᵘə xa tʂɛ

book 3rd-POSS break RES MOD-PART

'His book got torn up.'

In (12), the suffix nə refers to the subject of the sentence, meaning "my own home". The suffix ɳ̩i closely following a noun indicates "his". In Dongxiang as in other Mongolic languages, this slot can be filled by mini (my), ʧini (your) and ni (his). We will not give more examples in this paper due to space limitations. Be aware that this kind of suffix has been completely absorbed by those Tangwang people who now self-identify as Muslim. The source of these suffixes is actually the Dongxiang language (Chart 3).

It is useful to know that the Dongxiang language has simplified the reflexive suffixes compared to Mongolian, which possesses four forms due to vowel harmony. Only nə is attested in Dongxiang, and the Tangwang language has copied the same use. As for possessive suffixes, the Tangwang language has only borrowed the 3rd person form from the Dongxiang language, which has three forms just like in other Mongolian dialects.

Another suffix attested in all Mongolic languages is the terminative [thala], which has different phonetic forms due to vowel harmony, and expresses "until". One example from Tangwang:

(14) ɳ̩i pa ʨiɛ̃ thala ʦu ma tʂɛ

2SG eight o'clock TERM do what INTER

'What are you doing until 8 o'clock?'

This suffix is frequently attested in Gansu-Qinghai Sinitic languages even though the neighboring languages are quite different. Qinghai is more strongly influenced by Amdo Tibetan and Gansu by Mongolic languages. Compared with Thomason and Kaufman's borrowing scale, the language of Tangwang already presents some features of the highest degree of borrowing. Can we then confirm that the Tangwang language is a "mixed language"?

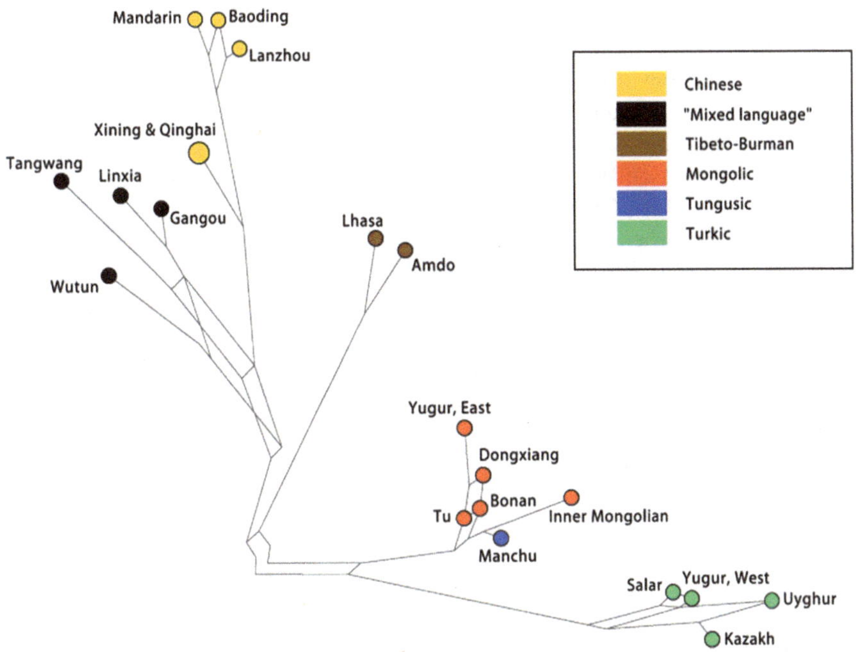

Fig. 4 Classification of different languages with 96 linguistic features

How can linguists measure the degree of typological change? Can we quantify the changes that occur due to language contact? In this study we have tried to find a more reliable method to face these problems encountered by many linguists. First of all, we have chosen 11 languages in the Sino-Tibetan family and 10 languages in the Altaic family. These two language families cover our target region, the border between Gansu and Qinghai. 96 linguistic features have been selected including 39 phonetic, phonological and morphological criteria, and 57 syntactic features. We have made all of these language features computable, converting them into a binary system. In this way the research will be based on algorithmic statistics instead of on experience-like studies. Here is the result of the work in a form which is easier to visualize (Fig. 4).

Some comments are necessary. Most of these languages are presented in four major groups (branches). What is interesting is that the Tangwang language undoubtedly clusters with the Sinitic group but not at all with Tibetan group, nor with the Altaic language family branch. This is also the case for Linxia, Gangou and Wutun languages. Before calculating these statistics, the Wutun and Tangwang languages were expected to be an isolated subgroup. But the chart shows the opposite. The Linxia language is still considered a Chinese dialect, while the status of Gangou has not been clearly defined. However the Wutun language is openly categorized as a mixed language (Sun et al. [eds.] 2007) by Chinese linguists. Nevertheless the authors of *Wutun* (Janhunen et al. 2008: 7) consider that "Wutun has occasionally been quoted as an example of a ‘mixed’ language, perhaps even an actual ‘creole’. We know today that it is best classified as an independent and highly aberrant variety of Northwest Mandarin”. The situation in Wutun is actually rather complex and requires its own discussion (Xu forthcoming). Based only on linguistic criteria, Xu (2014) has also declared that the Tangwang language is a Chinese variety but not yet a “mixed language”. The group consisting of Wutun, Tangwang, Linxia and Gangou form a sub-group of the main trunk of the Sinitic language group. Generally speaking, members of the Sino-Tibetan family appear less closely linked together than those of the Altaic family. In the latter, it is clear that the Turkic group shows a higher affinity between different languages than Mongolic group.

In conclusion, the Tangwang language, like Linxia, Gangou, may be considered a Chinese variety instead of a mixed language or creolized language. We do not mean to imply that our method can resolve all problems with criteria for classifying languages, but quantified data is always better than intuitive, experimental data.

6 Conclusion

Since the 1950s, and especially over the past few decades, language contact research has begun to draw the attention of many linguists, while the field of molecular biology only started developing in the 1980s. Since Cavalli-Sforza’s series of articles, geneticists and linguists have joined their efforts to establish and improve genetic and linguistic trees to better understand their correlations. It is taken for granted now that human languages and genes are correlated in most parts on the planet. However, this parallelism is broken in several parts of the Gansu-Qinghai area. This situation is reflected in the dispersal of small language units on the Hexi corridor. In this paper, we have tried to trace back the origins of these people to better understand their language.

All research requires approaches of varying scale, ranging from microscopic to macroscopic. Progress in human sciences research must be informed by other disciplines; efforts from different fields are required in order to break any new ground. This viewpoint reveals much room for improvement in the human sciences, and many avenues ripe for advancement. Combining linguistic and archaeological evidence, for example, might lead us to a new way of understanding the history of different peoples and their languages.

A comparison of language distance with ethnic genetic distance can help us to reconstruct the spread of different languages by dispersed populations, having diverse genes, over different historical periods. Such a comparison leads us to the question of why there are matches and mismatches in language-gene correlations at certain points in time and in certain locations. This sort of combination of natural sciences with human sciences lets us move beyond the limitations of traditional diachronic linguistic methodology.

Acknowledgements The authors of this paper express their thanks to Yao Hongbing and Wang Hua in helping Wen Shaoqing with sample collection in Tangwang, to Zhang Menghan for his statistics propositions and discussions, and to those who performed digitization: Saiyinjiya Caidengduoerji (for Mongolic languages and Manchu), Li Ting (for Tibetan languages), Barbara Kozhevina (for Turkic languages), Liu Keyou, and Wang Cong (for Sinitic languages).

References

Cavalli-Sforza, Luigi Luca, et al. 1994. *The History and Geography of Human Genes*. Princeton: Princeton University Press.

Cavalli-Sforza, Luigi Luca. 2000. *Gene, Peoples and Languages*. London: Penguin Group.

Chen, Naixiong. 1989. Wutun hua de dongci xingtai [Verbal morphology in Wutun]. *Minzu Yuwen* 6: 26–37.

Chen, Qiguang. 1999. Tonal accent in the Hezhou dialect. *Journal of the Linguistic Society of China* 9: 249–265.

Chen, Yuanlong. [A. Ibrahim] 1985. Gansu jingnei Tangwang hua jilüe [Sketch of Tangwang in Gansu province]. *Minzu Yuwen* 6: 33–47.

Cheng, Xianghui. 1980. Qinghai kouyu yufa sanlun [Essay on spoken grammar in Qinghai speech]. *Zhongguo Yuwen* 2: 143–149.

Daobu. 2007. Mengu yuzu [Mongolic languages]. In *Languages of China*, ed. Sun Hongkai et al., 1812–1820. Beijing: Shangwu yinshuguan.

Dwyer, Arienne M. 1992. Altaic Elements in the Linxia dialect: Contact-Induced Change on the Yellow River Plateau. *Journal of Chinese Linguistics* 20 (1): 160–178.

Janhunen, Juna 2004. [Abstract.] On the hierarchy of structural convergence in the Amdo Sprachbund. The Typology of Argument Structure and Grammatical Relations. *LENCA* 2. *Proceedings*, 70–72. Kazan'.

Janhunen, Juha, Peltomaa Marja, Sandman Erika, and Xiawu Dongzhou. 2008. *Wutun*. Muenchen: Lincom Europa.

Jia, Xiru. 1991. Qinghai hanhua yu shaoshu minzu yuyan [Chinese and minority languages in Qinghai]. *Minzu Yuwen* 5: 5–12.

Jia, Xiru. 1994. Cong Qinghai hanyu de jige fangyan ci kan yuyan jian de jiechu yingxiang. [Impact of language contact through some words in Qinghai dialect]. *Minzu Yuwen* 4: 57–63.

Karafet, T.M., et al. 2008. New binary polymorphisms reshape and increase resolution of the human Y chromosomal haplogroup tree. *Genome Research* 18 (5): 830–8.

Lanzhou Daxue zhongwenxi Linxia fangyan diaocha yanjiuzu, Gansu sheng Linxiazhou wenlian [the Linxia dialect research group of the Department of Chinese at Lanzhou University and Federation of Literary and Arts in Linxia, Gansu Province]. 1996. *Linxia fangyan [Dialects of Linxia]*. Lanzhou: Lanzhou daxue chubanshe.

Li, Charles N. 1983. Languages in contact in western China. *Papers in East Asian Languages* 1: 31–51.

Lin, Tao. 2009. Comparative studies on Shaanxi and Gansu phonetics in Central Asia. *Journal of Xianyang Normal University* 3: 44–47.

Liu, Lili. 1989. *Huimin Wulumuqi yuyan zhi* [Annals of Hui languages in Urumqi]. Urumqi: Xinjiang renmin chubanshe.

Liu, Zhaoxiong. 1981. *Dongxiangyu jianzhi [Outline of the Dongxiang Grammar]*. Beijing: Minzu chubanshe.

Luo, Peng. 2004. Hezhou hua yufa-yuyan jiechu de jieguo [The grammar of Hezhou speech—the result of language contact]. *Xibei Shida Xuebao* 4: 30–32.

Ma, Shujun. 1982. Linxia hua zhong de "ming + ha" jiegou ["Noun + ha" structures in Linxia dialect]. *Zhongguo Yuwen* 1: 72–73.

Ma, Shujun. 1984. Hanyu Hezhou hua yu A'ertai yuyan [Hezhou dialect and Altaic languages]. *Minzu Yuwen* 2: 50–55.

Peyraube, Alain. 2014. A comparative analysis of the case system in some Northwestern Sinitic languages. (Paper first presented at Workshop on language contact. Beijing, September 2009). In *Languages in contact in Northwestern China* ed. Cao, Djamouri and Peyraube, 191–125. Paris: Monograph series of the CRLAO.

Qi, X. et al. 2013. Genetic evidence of paleolithic colonization and neolithic expansion of modern humans on the tibetan plateau. *Molecular Biology and Evolution.* August 30(8):1761–1778.

Ren, Bisheng. 2004. Xining fangyan de qianzhi binyuju [Preverbal object structures in Xining dialect]. *Fangyan* 4: 338–346.

Shi, H., et al. 2008. Y chromosome evidence of earliest modern human settlement in East Asia and multiple origins of Tibetan and Japanese populations. *BMC Biology* 6: 45.

Sun, Hongkai, Hu Zengyi, and Huang Xing (eds.). 2007. *Zhongguo de yuyan [Languages of China].* Beijing: Shangwu yinshuguan.

Tang, Hanqing. 1987. *Huigu tongnian shidai Tangwang chuan.* [Memoirs of Tangwang in my childhood], [manuscript].

Tang, Zhi. 2011. *Tangwang shehuishi zhuanti yanjiu* [Studies of social history in Tangwang]. Master thesis.

Thomason, Sarah Grey, and Kaufman Terrence. 1988. *Language Contact, Creolization, and Genetic Linguistics.* Berkeley/Los Angeles: University of California Press.

Wang, Chuanchao, et al. 2012. Present Y chromosomes reveal the ancestry of Emperor Cao Cao of 1800 years ago. *Journal of Human Genetics* 57: 216–218.

Wang, Chuan-Chao et al. 2013. Late Neolithic expansion of ancient Chinese revealed by Y chromosome haplogroup O3a1c-002611. *Journal of Systematics and Evolution* (Special Issue of Human and Human-influenced Evolution) 51(3): 280–286.

Wang, Chuan-Chao, et al. 2014. Genetic structure of Qiangic populations residing in the Western Sichuan corridor. *PLoS ONE* 9 (8): e103772.

Wang, Chuanchao, and Li Hui. 2013. Inferring Human History in East Asia from Y Chromosomes. *Investigative Genetics* 4: 11.

Wang, Peiji, and Wu Xinhua. 1981. Guanyu Qinghai kouyu yufa de ji ge wenti [Some problems on the vernacular grammar of Qinghai dialect]. *Zhongguo Yuwen* 1: 50–53.

Wang, Sen. 1993. Gansu Linxia fangyan de liangzhong yuxu [Two word orders in Linxia dialect in Gansu]. *Fangyan* 3: 191–194.

Wang, William.S.-Y. 2000. Linguistic diversity and language relationships. In *New Horizons in Chinese Linguistics*, ed. C.-T. James Huang and Yen-hui Audrey Li, 235–267. Dordrecht: Kluwer Academic Publishers.

Weinreich, Uriel. 1968. *[1953: originally published as Number 1 in the series "Publications of the Linguistic Circle of New York] Languages in Contact-Findings and Problems.* The Hague: Mouton de Gruyter.

Xu, Dan. 2011. *Tangwang hua de ge biaoji* [Case marking in Tangwang]. *Zhongguo Yuwen* 2: 145–154.

Xu, Dan. 2014. *Tangwang hua yanjiu* [Studies of the Tangwang language] Beijing: Minzu chubanshe.

Xu, Dan. 2015a. Tangwang Initials. In *Languages in contact in Northwestern China* ed. Cao et al. ed., 319–338. Paris: Monograph series of the EHESS-CRLAO.

Xu, Dan. 2015b. Sinitic languages of Northwest China: Where did their case marking come from? In *Languages in contact in Northwestern China*, Cao et al. eds., 217–244 Paris: Monograph series of the EHESS-CRLAO.

Xu, Dan, Wen Shaoqing, and Xie Xiaodong. 2013. The Dongxiang language and people. *Journal of Cambridge Studies* 8 (2): 40–48.

Yan, Shi, et al. 2014. Y chromosomes of 40% Chinese descend from three Neolithic super-grandfathers. *PLoS ONE* 9 (8): e105691.

Zerjal, T., et al. 2003. The genetic legacy of the Mongols. *The American Journal of Human Genetics* 72: 717–721.

Zhang, Chengcai. 2006. *Zhonggu yin yu Qinghai fangyin zihui* [Middle Chinese pronunciation and vocabulary in Qinghai dialects] Xining: Qinghai renmin chubanshe.

Zhangjiacun zhi [Annals of the Zhang family]. 2004. *Authors unknown*. Lanzhou: Gansu Xintong yinwu youxian zeren gongsi.

Zhong, H., et al. 2010. Global distribution of Y-chromosome haplogroup C reveals the prehistoric migration routes of African exodus and early settlement. *East Asia. Journal of Human Genetics* 55: 428–435.

Zhu, Yongzhong, Chuluu Üjiyediin, Slater Keith, and Stuart Kevin. 1997. Gangou Chinese Dialect-A Comparative Study of a Strongly Altaicized Chinese Dialect and Its Mongolic Neighbor. *Anthropos* 92: 433–450.

Present Y Chromosomes Refute the Roma/Gypsy Origin of the Xuejiawan People in Northwest China

Shaoqing Wen, Dan Xu, Hongbing Yao and Hui Li

1 Introduction

Northwestern China is rich in human genetic and linguistic resources. Notably, it is here that the ancient Silk Road snaked from its eastern terminus in Xi'an across the mountains and deserts to the West, leaving behind a number of ethnic groups with different religious faiths, cultures and customs due to East-West intercommunications. Early in 1947, the Chinese journalist Zhu Tian proposed that the Xuejiawan people in Yongdeng County, once an important town on the ancient Silk Road, were eastern Gypsies (Zhu 1947). Thereafter, compared to the neighboring Han farmers, this special population who has made their living mainly by fortune-telling has generated enormous publicity. So far, dozens of articles have been published discussing the ethnic origins of the Xuejiawan people from various perspectives (Tuo 2006; Yang 1991; Wu et al. 2001; Wu 1990, 1991; Guan and Zhang 2012). Based on folkloric and historic comparisons, some scholars hold the ancient Gypsy

S. Wen (✉)
MOE Key Laboratory of Contemporary Anthropology, School of Life Sciences, Fudan University, Shanghai 200433, People's Republic of China
e-mail: wenshaoqing1982@gmail.com

S. Wen · D. Xu
Institut National des Langues et Civilisations Orientales (INALCO), 63 Rue des Grands Moulins, 75013 Paris, France

D. Xu
CRLAO (CNRS), Paris, France

H. Yao
Key Laboratory of Evidence Science of Gansu Province, Gansu Institute of Political Science and Law, Lanzhou 730070, People's Republic of China

H. Li
MOE Key Laboratory of Contemporary Anthropology, School of Life Sciences, Fudan University, Shanghai 200438, People's Republic of China

D. Xu and H. Li (eds.), *Languages and Genes in Northwestern China and Adjacent Regions*, DOI 10.1007/978-981-10-4169-3_7

origin hypothesis, i.e. that the Xuejiawan people were the descendents of gypsies who appeared in China in the Yuan Dynasty (Yang 1991) or Qing Dynasty (Zhu 1947). Others support the native Chinese origin hypothesis, which is further divided into two alternative hypotheses, the southern Hmong-Mien and Han Chinese origin hypotheses. The former was propounded on the basis of incomplete lexical comparison (Wu et al. 2001), while the latter was presented based on local historical anthropologists' long-term fieldwork (Wu 1990, 1991; Guan and Zhang 2012). Among these hypotheses, the Gypsy origin hypothesis is the most famous as the exotic image it creates caters to popular taste. A best-selling novel, *Belly Drum*, was written to vividly reflect the imaginative history and real experiences of these so-called Eastern Gypsies. Like DNA, some cultural items such as language are normally transmitted from parents to offspring (Pagel 2009). Therefore, when lacking written records, current genetic and linguistic data can be used to trace the ancestry information of a subject population (Hunley et al. 2008; Balanovsky et al. 2011; Karafet et al. 2016). Here, to address the questions of the ethnic origin and population history of the Xuejiawan people, we, a joint team formed by Chinese geneticists and French linguists, performed an interdisciplinary investigation in Xuejiawan village, focusing on a wide-ranging comparison of paternal lineages and word lists.

2 Materials and Methods

2.1 Subjects

According to the local chronicles, there are four representative clans of Xuejiawan people, Liú (刘), Liǔ (柳), Gao (高) and Hé (何), accounting for the bulk of the population. The rest, such as Hao (郝) and Guo (郭), are minor clans. Accordingly, we collected oral samples of 118 healthy male individuals from six clans, including 31 individuals with the surname Liú (刘), 39 with Liǔ (柳), 30 with Gao (高), 15 with He (何), 2 with Hao (郝), and 1 with Guo (郭), in Xuejiawan village, Yongdeng County, Gansu Province (Fig. 1). This study was approved by the Ethics Committee for Biological Research at Fudan University, and all the samples were collected with informed consent.

2.2 Genetic Data

Genomic DNA was extracted using DP-318 Kit (Tiangen Biotechnology, Beijing), and Y chromosomes were characterized using two marker systems of different mutability. Initially, we amplified 17 Y-STRs (DYS19, DYS389I/II, DYS390, DYS391, DYS392, DYS393, DYS437, DYS438, DYS439, DYS448, DYS456, DYS458, DYS635, Y-GATA H4, DYS385a/b) using Y-Filer kit (Life Technologies,

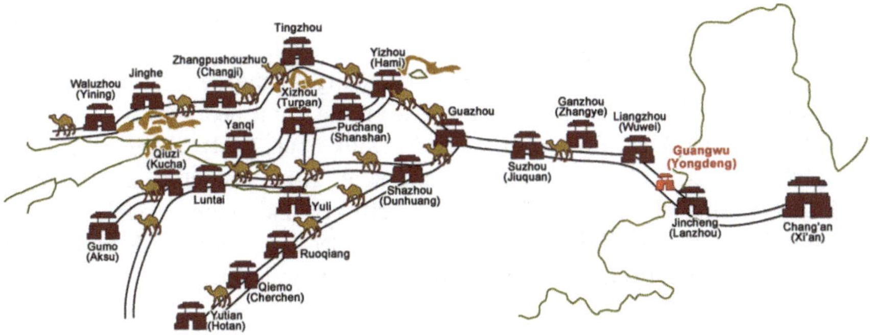

Fig. 1 The Xuejiawan village is located in Yongdeng County, which was once called Guangwu County in Tang Dynasty, an important town on the ancient Silk Road

CA, USA). Moreover, using a hierarchical genotyping strategy, we first genotyped phylogenetically relevant Y-chromosomal SNPs as listed in the latest Y-chromosomal tree described in previous studies (Wang et al. 2014). The O3a1c*-002611 and O3a2c1*-M134+,M117- individuals were then genotyped respectively by two panels successfully used in our previous studies (Wang et al. 2013a; Ning et al. 2016). According to the inferred SNP haplogroups of each sample via our private Y-chromosome database, the C3*-M217 individuals were then subjected to further typing of six biallelic markers, F1067, F2613, F1396, F6733/FGC16362, F3918, F1756, using SNaPshot multiplex kit (ABI, Carlsbad, California, US).

2.3 *Linguistic Data*

We carried out an investigation of the Xuejiawan language, covering varied aspects of phonology and morpho-syntax. Because the Xuejiawan language faces extinction, we tried to retrieve as much linguistic information as possible. In particular, about 400 words were collected.

3 Statistical Analysis

Networks of Y chromosomal STR data were constructed by the reduced median-joining method using NETWORK v. 5.0.0.0 (Fluxus-engineering.com). Notably, except for two lineages (O3a1c1-F11 and O3a1c2-F238) which were constructed based on ten Y-STR loci (DYS19, DYS389I, DYS389II, DYS390, DYS391, DYS392, DYS393, DYS437, DYS438, and DYS439), the networks for the remaining five lineages employed 15 STRs data (excluding DYS385a and DYS385b). Time estimations for each Y-chromosomal lineage in the Xuejiawan people were made by ASD and BATWING methods as we did before (Wang et al. 2014; Wang and Li 2015), assuming a generation time of 25 years. Reference population data on the Y chromosomes belonging to the detected haplogroups found in Xuejiawan people were retrieved from the published reports (Kim et al. 2011; Haber et al. 2012; Roewer et al. 2007; Dulik et al. 2011; Abilev et al. 2012; Zhaxylyk et al. 2012; Cai et al. 2011; Wang et al. 2014; Yan et al. 2011; Trejaut et al. 2014; Ning et al. 2016; Wang et al. 2013a), and some unpublished data including Han Chinese, Hui, Yugur, Dongxiang, Baonan, Kazakh, Mongolian and Tibetan were drawn from our lab's database (Wang et al. 2015).

4 Genetic Structure of the Xuejiawan People

According to the nomenclature of the Y Chromosome Consortium (Yan et al. 2011, 2014; Karafet et al. 2008), seven paternal lineages were determined from the 118 individual Xuejiawan samples (Fig. 2 and Table S1). Haplogroup C3-M217 gave rise to two downstream haplogroups, a southern clade (C3-S) defined by F1067, especially frequent in Han Chinese, and a northern clade (C3-N) defined by F1396, prevalent in Altaic-speaking populations (Yan et al. 2014). C3-S-F2613+,M407-, derived from the southern clade, was quite common in northern Han Chinese, 14.29 and 9.87% in Northeastern and Northern Han, respectively (Zhong et al. 2010; our unpublished data), and was only found with moderate frequency in the Liú (刘) clan (12.9%). C3-N-F1756 derived from the northern clade, whose STR haplotypes display the null allele at DYS448 (Park et al. 2012), was a brother haplogroup of C3* star-cluster, a famous paternal lineage associated with Genghis Khan (Zerjal et al. 2003). C3-N-F1756 was commonly seen in Kazakhstan (Kazakhs, 11.11%), Hailar in Inner Mongolia (Mongolian, 9.26%) and the Altai Republic in Russia (Altain, 12.50%; Teleuts, 9.09%), but was absent or found with very low frequency in Han Chinese (Zhong et al. 2010; our unpublished data). This subclade was exclusively detected with high frequency (94.87%) in the Liǔ (柳) clan. The basal O2*-M268+,PK4- containing Emperor Cao Cao's paternal lineage (Wang et al. 2012, 2013b), which was abundant in Northern and Eastern parts of China, accounts for about 5% of the Han Chinese (Yan et al. 2011). In this study, it was detected once in the Liǔ (柳) clan, represents about half of the Y chromosomes observed in He (何) clan, and reaches the highest frequency in the Gao (高) clan (100%), showing a common descent from a single paternal ancestor. O3a1c-002611, O3a2c1*-M134 and O3a2c1a-M117, three main subclades of O3-M122 were seen as the three super-grandfathers of about 40% of modern Chinese (Yan et al. 2014). According to the east-to-west pattern of phylogeographic distribution, O3a2c1*-M134 and O3a2c1a-M117 exhibit high frequencies in northern Han Chinese and Tibeto-Burman populations, whereas O3a1c-002611 is more frequent in the eastern Han Chinese (Wang et al. 2013a, 2014). In the Xuejiawan people, O3a2c1a-M117 and O3a2c1*-M134 were exclusively detected in the Liú (刘) clan at high (70.97%) and moderate levels (16.13%), respectively.

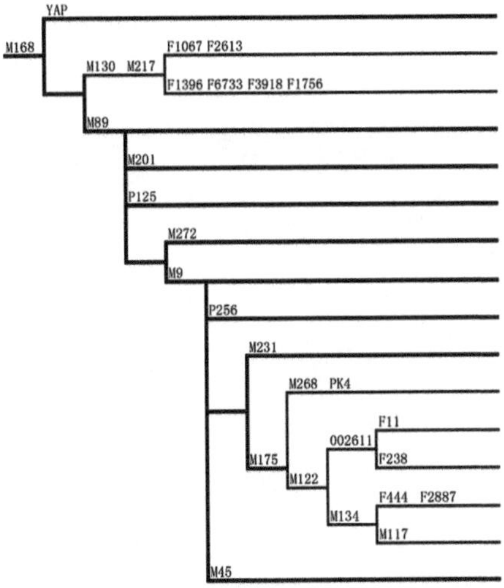

Clan	Liu 刘	Liu 柳	Gao 高	He 何	Hao 郝	Guo 郭
Sample size	31	39	30	15	2	1
(DE)	-	-	-	-	-	-
C3-S-F2613+, M407-	12.90	-	-	-	-	-
C3-N-F1756	-	94.87	-	-	-	-
(F)	-	-	-	-	-	-
(G)	-	-	-	-	-	-
(IJ)	-	-	-	-	-	-
(T)	-	-	-	-	-	-
(K)	-	-	-	-	-	-
(M)	-	-	-	-	-	-
(N)	-	-	-	-	-	-
O2*-M268+, PK4-, M176-	-	2.56	100.00	53.00	-	-
O3a1c1-F11	-	2.56	-	47.00	-	100.00
O3a1c2-F238	-	-	-	-	100.00	-
O3a2c1*-F2887	16.13	-	-	-	-	-
O3a2c1a-M117	70.97	-	-	-	-	-
(P)	-	-	-	-	-	-

Fig. 2 The phylogenetic relationship of Y-chromosome haplogroups surveyed in this study and their clan-based frequencies among the Xuejiawan people. The marker names are shown along the branches, and haplogroup names are shown on the *right side*. Potentially paraphyletic undefined subgroups are distinguished from recognized haplogroups by the *asterisk* symbol. Haplogroups tested for but not seen in this study are enclosed in parentheses

O3a1c1-F11, one subclade of O3a1c-002611, was observed at considerable frequencies in the He (何) clan (47%), and was separately observed once in Liǔ (柳) clan and Guo (郭) clan. O3a1c2-F238, a brother subclade of O3a1c1-F11, was only found in Hao (郝). In summary, the dominant paternal lineages in various clans have a definite East Asian origin, for instance C3-S-F2613+,M407-, O3a2c1*-F2887 and O3a2c1a-M117 in the Liú (刘) clan, C3-N-F1756 in the Liǔ (柳) clan, O2*-M268+,PK4-,M176- in the Gao (高) clan, O2*-M268+,PK4-,M176- and O3a1c1-F11 in the He (何) clan, O3a1c2-F238 in the Hao (郝) clan and O3a1c1-F11 in the Guo (郭) clan.

5 Network Analysis and Time Estimation

To discern the detailed relationships between seven East Asian lineages in the Xuejiawan people and other related populations, median-joining networks constructed based on Y-STR haplotypes of those haplogroups were shown in Fig. 3 and Doc S1. In the network C3-N-F1756, 24 Liǔ (柳) clan individuals rooted in the central zone were shared by a northern Han individual, and were closely related with the remaining Liǔ (柳) clan individuals and the individuals from northwestern

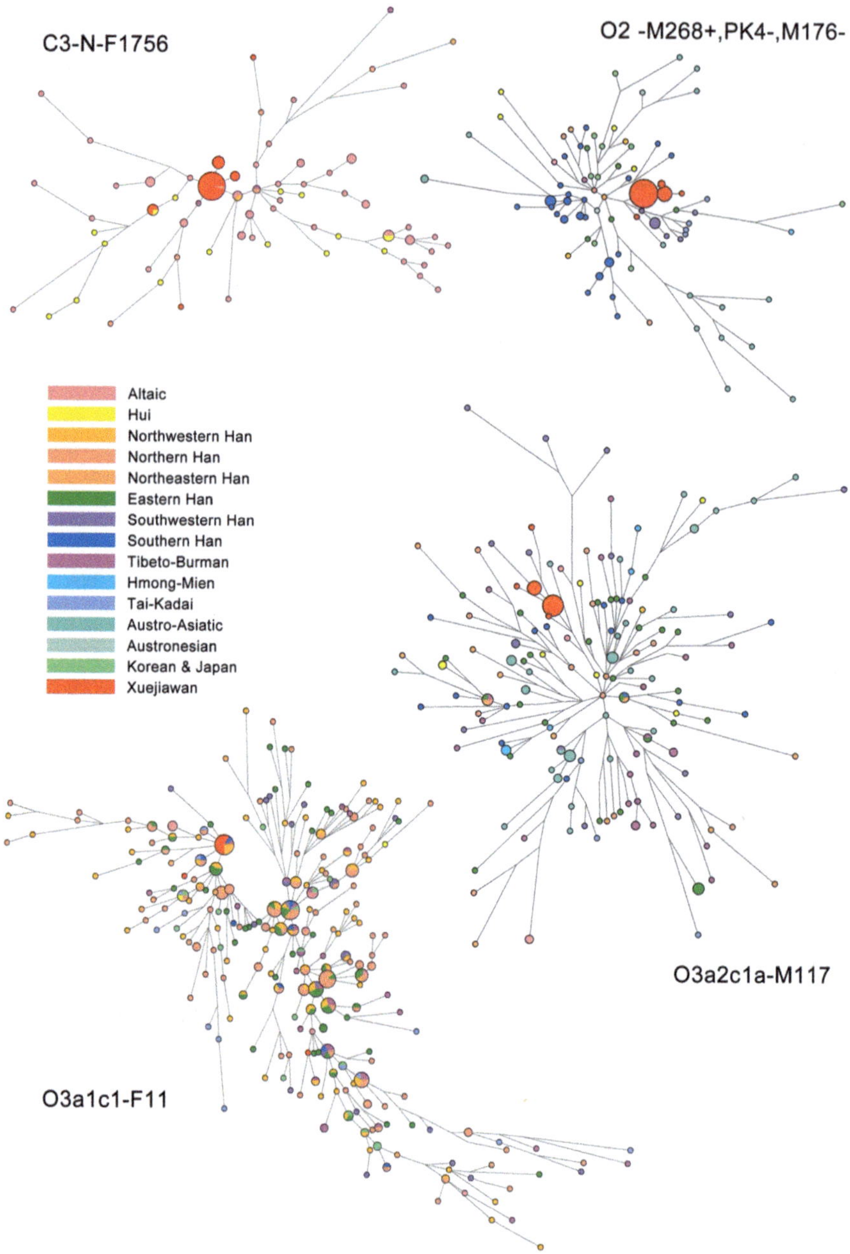
C3-N-F1756
O2 -M268+,PK4-,M176-
Altaic
Hui
Northwestern Han
Northern Han
Northeastern Han
Eastern Han
Southwestern Han
Southern Han
Tibeto-Burman
Hmong-Mien
Tai-Kadai
Austro-Asiatic
Austronesian
Korean & Japan
Xuejiawan
O3a2c1a-M117
O3a1c1-F11

◂**Fig. 3** Median-joining networks of Y-STR haplotypes for the four dominant haplogroup lineages (C3-N-F1756, O2*-M268+,PK4-,M176-, O3a1c1-F11 and O3a2c1a-M117) in the Xuejiawan people. Haplotypes are represented by circles with area proportional to the number of individuals. Colors indicate geographic origin. Notably, northwestern Han refers to the ethnic Han individuals originating from the provinces of Shaanxi, Gansu and Xinjiang; northern Han refers to Hebei, Henan, Shandong, Shanxi, Tianjin and Beijing; northeastern Han refers to Jilin, Liaoning, Heilongjiang and Inner Mongolia; eastern Han refers to Jiangsu, Jiangxi, Zhejiang, Anhui and Shanghai; southern Han refers to Guangdong, Hainan, Hunan, Hubei and Fujian; southwestern Han refers to Yunnan, Chongqing, Guangxi, Guizhou and Sichuan

populations, especially Kazakhs, Gansu Hui and Shaanxi Han, implying a native northwestern Chinese origin of Liǔ (柳) clan. A clear Xuejiawan-specific cluster comprising one Liǔ (柳) clan, eight He (何) clan and 30 Gao (高) clan individuals can be identified from the O2*-M268+,PK4-,M176- network, which was located on the branch mainly containing Pinghua populations in Southwestern China, suggesting a common descent from a single ancestor and a tie between the O2*-M268+, PK4-,M176- individuals in Xuejiawan people and the Southwestern Chinese populations. In the upper part of the O3a1c1-F11 network, a cluster contained one Liǔ (柳) clan, seven He (何) clan individuals and some Northwestern and Northern Han individuals, and demonstrated a star-like pattern with a central founder haplotype and a few subfounders. Notably, the Guo (郭) clan individuals belonged to a different cluster in the lower part of the network, revealing a different origin. The Liú (刘) clan individuals were found in a small cluster in the upper part of the O3a1c1-F11 network, which mainly comprises Pinghua populations in Southwestern China. Reduced median networks for the remaining lineages, O3a2c1a-M117, C3-S-F2613+,M407-, O3a1c2-F238 and O3a2c1*-F2887 (Doc S1), displayed similar patterns of branching. Accordingly, the 22 Liú (刘) clan individuals and northwestern Han individuals formed a unique cluster, the four Liú (刘) clan individuals were much closer to northern Han individuals, the two Hao (郝) clan individuals were clustered with northwestern Han and northern Han individuals, and the five Liú (刘) clan individuals showed a close genetic relationship with eastern Han individuals.

Having inferred the putative origins of the clan-based Y chromosomal lineages in the Xuejiawan people at individual level, we then estimated the coalescence time for each paternal lineage using both the ASD and BATWING methods (Table 1 and Table S2). In our previous case studies evaluating Y-STR dating in deep-rooted pedigrees, we found that the Y-chromosomal genealogical mutation rates (OMRB and lmMR) in the BATWING method can give the best-fit estimation for historical lineage dating (Wang and Li 2015). Hence, in the Xuejiawan people, four paternal lineages, O3a2c1a-M117, C3a1-F2613+,M407-, C3-N-F1756, and O3a1c1-F11, can trace their common ancestor to the Tang and Song dynasties. The coalescence of subhaplogroup O2*-M268+,PK4-,M176- was more likely in the late Yuan and early Ming Dynasties. Because they share a Y chromosomal haplotype, the lineages O3a2c1*-F2887 and O3a1c2-F238 cannot be meaningfully used for Y-STR dating, suggesting that their coalescence times were quite recent.

Table 1 The partial results of coalescence time estimations for each paternal lineage in the Xuejiawan people using BATWING (time in years)

Haplogroup	Clan	Putative origins	lmMR		OMRB		Period
			TMRCA	95% CI	TMRCA	95% CI	
O2*-M268+,PK4-,M176-	Gao	Southwest	504.4	59.4-3455.9	474.4	55.7-3265.4	Ming Dynasty
	He	Southwest	559	33.5-6286.8	534.7	32.1-5998.1	Ming Dynasty
O3a2c1a-M117	Liú	Northwest	977.6	157.5-5764.4	945.2	151.5-5641.1	Song Dynasty
C3-S-F2613+,M407-	Liú	North	1093.4	48.7-17359.2	1066	46.3-17172.1	Song Dynasty
O3a2c1*-F2887	Liú	East	–	–	–	–	Recent times
C3-N-F1756	Liǔ	Northwest	1181	208.3-6520	1140.9	199.9-6356.7	Five Dynasties
O3a1c1-F11	He	Northwest/North	1332.9	133.2-11387.7	1283.8	127.9-10987.8	Tang Dynasty
	Guo	Northwest	–	–	–	–	Recent times
O3a1c2-F238	Hao	Northwest/North	–	–	–	–	Recent times

6 Linguistic Affinity of the Xuejiawan Language

The Xuejiawan language is phonetically similar to Yongdeng dialect, which belongs to the Jincheng group of Lanyin Mandarin. Additionally, compared to Northwestern Chinese dialects, the Xuejiawan language has some specific phonetic features. Firstly, in addition to its front-back nasal merger like the surrounding Chinese dialects, the Xuejiawan language sometimes leaves out the nasal element, such as pronounting today (今闲) as ʨi^{11}ɕiɛ^{13} (allophones of ʨĩ^{11}ɕiɛ̃^{13}) and woman (娘娘) as ȵia ȵia (instead of ȵiã ȵiã). Secondly, plosives and fricatives/affricates, as well as fricatives and affricates, can sometimes be pronounced interchangeably without misunderstanding; for instance, both tĩ^{11} kuɛ^{33} and ɕĩ^{11} kuɛ^{13} mean 'thing' (东西), liu^{11} thĩ^{31} and liu^{11} ʨhĩ^{31} mean 'kerchief' (头巾), phiɛ^{13} suə^{31} and phiɛ^{13} tsuə^{31} mean 'cry/blow' (哭,吹) etc. Syntactically, the Xuejiawan language is grouped with Sinitic languages rather than with minority languages. Some nearby Chinese dialects in Gansu province, such as Hezhou, Tangwang and Xining, have changed their word order from SVO (subject-verb-object) to SOV (subject-object-verb), being affected by surrounding Altaic languages. However, the Xuejiawan language has kept the word order SVO, which is common in all Chinese dialects. Interestingly, the Xuejiawan language has a peculiar pronoun system [e.g. xə^{11}ʨhĩ^{33} (贺秦) means 'I/me', ʨhĩ^{11} ʨia^{33} (秦家) designates 'you' and 'he/she'], the numeral system (e.g. lio^{33} tʂə^{11} ʦɿ 'one', mi^{11} tʂə^{33} ʦɿ 'two', etc.) and interrogative system [e.g. WH question words are expressed with the same form nuo^{11}tu^{33} (挪都) or nə^{11}tuə^{13} (呢多)]. In a word, despite having its own characteristics, the Xuejiawan language unequivocally belongs to the Sinitic languages from phonetic and syntactic perspectives.

Then we must ask the question, what linguistic elements make the Xuejiawan language unintelligible for the peripheral Han farmers? In other words, how is the Xuejiawan language so different from the neighboring Chinese dialects? To address this issue, a word list containing 406 words from the Xuejiawan language has been dissected and compared with other potentially associated languages, including Altaic, Hmong and Chinese languages. Actually, the Xuejiawan people employed Chinese means of word formation. Among the 406 collected words, 318 words have been derived from gang languages of various historic periods, covering 13 words from the Song and Yuan dynasties, 10 words from the Ming and Qing Dynasties, 48 words from the end of the Qing Dynasty, and 247 words from the contemporary era; 55 words come from Northwestern Chinese dialect, 17 words from Swadesh's 200-word list have been lost by the Xuejiawan people, 6 words come from Altaic languages and the remaining 10 words could not be identified (Fig. 4).

On the one hand, 78.32% commonly used words in the Xuejiawan language are derived from various argots and some argot words can be dated back to the Song dynasty, making it hard for the neighboring Han farmers to understand. On the other hand, the Xuejiawan people have created many new words. This word-building rule is to create new words based on the limited existing vocabulary.

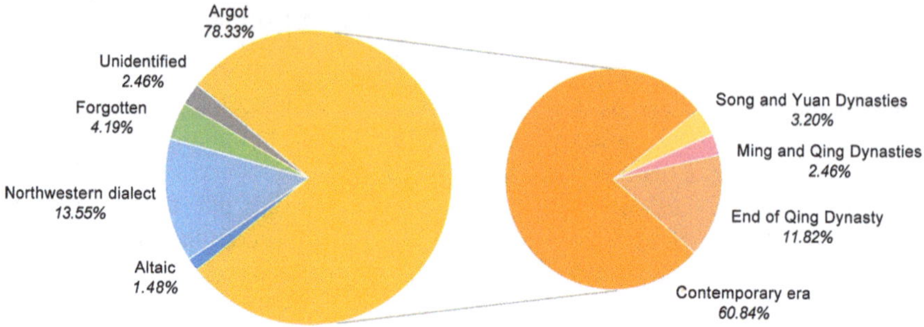

Fig. 4 The lexical composition of the Xuejiawan's 406 word-list

For example, sɿ^{33}ma^{11} (司马) means 'vehicle' (车) in the Xuejiawan language; subsequently, they created the new words xũ^{33} tsɿ^{31}sɿ^{33} ma^{11} (fire + vehicle, 红子司马), tɕiɛ̃^{13}sɿ^{33} ma^{31} (little + vehicle, 尖司马) and xe^{33} sɿ^{33}ma^{11}(big + vehicle 海司马), instead of saying 'train' (火车), 'bicycle' (自行车) and 'car' (大汽车), where the first syllables mean fire (火), small (小) and large (大), respectively. In addition, the Xuejiawan people sometimes assembled the existing words into a phrase in order to represent a new thing. For example, they put three words together, jũ^{33} tʂɑ^{31} ('water' 云掌), li (postposition like other Chinese dialects 'in' 里) and fa^{11} la^{33} ('to play' 耍拉), to express the meaning 'swimming'. Therefore, the unique argot words, as well as the created new words based on the extant vocabulary, have caused the public and some scholars to misunderstand the Xuejiawan language as a foreign language or minority language.

7 Discussion

The Roma (Gypsies), which represent a population of 10–15 million living throughout Europe and West Asia, have no nation-state, speak different languages, belong to many religions and comprise a mosaic of socially and culturally divergent endogamous groups (Kalaydjieva et al. 2005). Linguistically, the Gypsies speak more than 60 dialects called *Romani*, which are most closely related to the Northwestern Indian languages like Punjabi or Kashmiri or Central Indian languages like Hindi, suggesting an Indian origin of the Gypsies (Turner 1984). Previous genetic studies also supported the scenario that the Gypsies originated after their exodus from India about 1000–1500 years ago (Moorjani et al. 2013; Mendizabal et al. 2012; Gomez-Carballa et al. 2013). Y-chromosome haplogroup H1a1a-M82 (Kalaydjieva et al. 2001; Pamjav et al. 2011; Rai et al. 2012), mtDNA haplogroup M5a1, M18 and M35b (Mendizabal et al. 2011), and several disease-causing mutations (for instance, the congenital myasthenia 1267delG mutation) (Morar et al. 2004), found on the same ancestral chromosomal background in Gypsy, Indian and Pakistani subjects, has demonstrated a strong genetic link between the proto-Gypsies and Northwestern Indian. Furthermore, it is clear that, in the Romani paternal gene pool, Y-chromosomal lineages were from two different putative origins, ancestral Indian (H1a-M82) and later mixed present-day Eurasian (J2a2-M67, J2*-M172, E1b1b1a-M78, I1-M253, I2a-P37.2, R1a1-M198 and R1b1-P25) during their migration route (Zalan et al. 2011).

In this study, seven East Asian lineages assigned to two major clades C and O were found in the Xuejiawan people, definitively disproving the Gypsy origin hypothesis. Furthermore, due to the evidences from network analysis and lexical comparison, we found that the formation of the Xuejiawan people was a dynamic process and was mainly divided into three stages, albeit with some uncertainty: the mixing of paternal lineages O3a1c1-F11, C3-N-F1756, C3-S-F2613+,M407- and O3a2c1a-M117 in the Song dynasty when they might have primarily spoken Northern varieties; the participation of lineage O2*-M268+,PK4-,M176- in the late Yuan and early Ming Dynasties when some Southern vocabulary might have been introduced, and the immigration of lineages O3a2c1*-F2887 and O3a1c2-F238 in recent times as the Northwestern Chinese dialects have gradually expanded their influence on the Xuejiawan people.

With their nomadic lifestyle and endogamous social practices, the Xuejiawan people have been socially marginalized and historically persecuted in the past, resembling the same historical experiences of the Gypsies in the West. Coincidentally, the Xuejiawan people have chosen a means of living by fortune-telling, instead of farming. Therefore, the Xuejiawan people could be easily misinterpreted as Eastern Gypsies. In addition, they speak a language derived from the gang languages of various historic periods, emphasizing their mystique and thus meeting the demands of their vocation. There are two similar cases from elsewhere in the world, in which Uisai speakers in Papua New Guinea and Quechua speakers in Peru have changed the linguistic elements to make their language differ from the surrounding languages, due to various social and cultural causes (Thomason 2001, 2003).

Acknowledgements We thank all the volunteers and the local guide Xiaosheng Li for sample collection. This work was partly supported by NSFC for Excellent Young Scholars (31222030), MOE Scientific Research Project (113022A), the Shanghai Shuguang Project (14SG05), the French National Research Agency (No. ANR-12-BSH2-0004-01), the Natural Science Foundation of Gansu province (1308RJZA190), and the Scientific Research Project for Colleges of Gansu Province (2014A-085).

Supporting Information

Table S1. Y-chromosome SNP and STR data for the Xuejiawan people.

Table S2. The detailed results of coalescence time estimations for each paternal lineage in the Xuejiawan population using both BATWING and ASD methods (time in years).

Doc S1. Median-joining networks of Y-STR haplotypes for the remaining three paternal lineages (C3-S-F2613+,M407-, O3a1c2-F238 and O3a2c1*-F2887).

References

Abilev, S., B. Malyarchuk, M. Derenko, M. Wozniak, T. Grzybowski, and I. Zakharov. 2012. The Y-chromosome C3* star-cluster attributed to Genghis Khan's descendants is present at high frequency in the Kerey clan from Kazakhstan. *Human Biology* 84 (1): 79–89.

Balanovsky, O., K. Dibirova, A. Dybo, O. Mudrak, S. Frolova, E. Pocheshkhova, M. Haber, D. Platt, T. Schurr, W. Haak, M. Kuznetsova, M. Radzhabov, O. Balaganskaya, A. Romanov, T. Zakharova, H.D. Soria, P. Zalloua, S. Koshel, M. Ruhlen, C. Renfrew, R.S. Wells, C. Tyler-Smith, and E. Balanovska. 2011. Parallel evolution of genes and languages in the Caucasus region. *Molecular Biology and Evolution* 28 (10): 2905–2920.

Cai, X., Z. Qin, B. Wen, S. Xu, Y. Wang, Y. Lu, L. Wei, C. Wang, S. Li, X. Huang, L. Jin, and H. Li. 2011. Human migration through bottlenecks from Southeast Asia into East Asia during Last Glacial Maximum revealed by Y chromosomes. *PLoS ONE* 6 (8): e24282.

Dulik, M.C., L.P. Osipova, and T.G. Schurr. 2011. Y-chromosome variation in Altaian Kazakhs reveals a common paternal gene pool for Kazakhs and the influence of Mongolian expansions. *PLoS ONE* 6 (3): e17548.

Gomez-Carballa, A., J. Pardo-Seco, L. Fachal, A. Vega, M. Cebey, N. Martinon-Torres, F. Martinon-Torres, and A. Salas. 2013. Indian signatures in the westernmost edge of the European Romani diaspora: New insight from mitogenomes. *PLoS ONE* 8 (10): e75397.

Guan, S.X., and H. Zhang. 2012. The research and analysis into the nationality—Belonging of "Xuejiawan Fortune-teller". *Journal of Gansu Lianhe University: social Sciences* 28 (1): 81–85.

Haber, M., D.E. Platt, B.M. Ashrafian, S.C. Youhanna, D.F. Soria-Hernanz, B. Martinez-Cruz, B. Douaihy, M. Ghassibe-Sabbagh, H. Rafatpanah, M. Ghanbari, J. Whale, O. Balanovsky, R.S. Wells, D. Comas, C. Tyler-Smith, and P.A. Zalloua. 2012. Afghanistan's ethnic groups share a Y-chromosomal heritage structured by historical events. *PLoS ONE* 7 (3): e34288.

Hunley, K., M. Dunn, E. Lindstrom, G. Reesink, A. Terrill, M.E. Healy, G. Koki, F.R. Friedlaender, and J.S. Friedlaender. 2008. Genetic and linguistic coevolution in Northern Island Melanesia. *PLoS Genetics* 4 (10): e1000239.

Kalaydjieva, L., F. Calafell, M.A. Jobling, D. Angelicheva, P. de Knijff, Z.H. Rosser, M.E. Hurles, P. Underhill, I. Tournev, E. Marushiakova, and V. Popov. 2001. Patterns of inter- and intra-group genetic diversity in the Vlax Roma as revealed by Y chromosome and mitochondrial DNA lineages. *European Journal of Human Genetics* 9 (2): 97–104.

Kalaydjieva, L., B. Morar, R. Chaix, and H. Tang. 2005. A newly discovered founder population: The Roma/Gypsies. *BioEssays* 27 (10): 1084–1094.

Karafet, T.M., F.L. Mendez, M.B. Meilerman, P.A. Underhill, S.L. Zegura, and M.F. Hammer. 2008. New binary polymorphisms reshape and increase resolution of the human Y chromosomal haplogroup tree. *Genome Research* 18 (5): 830–838.

Karafet, T.M., K.B. Bulayeva, J. Nichols, O.A. Bulayev, F. Gurgenova, J. Omarova, L. Yepiskoposyan, O.V. Savina, B.H. Rodrigue, and M.F. Hammer. 2016. Coevolution of genes and languages and high levels of population structure among the highland populations of Daghestan. *Journal of Human Genetics* 61 (3): 181–191.

Kim, S.H., K.C. Kim, D.J. Shin, H.J. Jin, K.D. Kwak, M.S. Han, J.M. Song, W. Kim, and W. Kim. 2011. High frequencies of Y-chromosome haplogroup O2b-SRY465 lineages in Korea: A genetic perspective on the peopling of Korea. *Investigative Genetics* 2 (1): 10.

Mendizabal, I., C. Valente, A. Gusmao, C. Alves, V. Gomes, A. Goios, W. Parson, F. Calafell, L. Alvarez, A. Amorim, L. Gusmao, D. Comas, and M.J. Prata. 2011. Reconstructing the Indian origin and dispersal of the European Roma: A maternal genetic perspective. *PLoS ONE* 6 (1): e15988.

Mendizabal, I., O. Lao, U.M. Marigorta, A. Wollstein, L. Gusmao, V. Ferak, M. Ioana, A. Jordanova, R. Kaneva, A. Kouvatsi, V. Kucinskas, H. Makukh, A. Metspalu, M.G. Netea, R. de Pablo, H. Pamjav, D. Radojkovic, S.J. Rolleston, J. Sertic, M.J. Macek, D. Comas, and M. Kayser. 2012. Reconstructing the population history of European Romani from genome-wide data. *Current Biology* 22 (24): 2342–2349.

Moorjani, P., N. Patterson, P.R. Loh, M. Lipson, P. Kisfali, B.I. Melegh, M. Bonin, L. Kadasi, O. Riess, B. Berger, D. Reich, and B. Melegh. 2013. Reconstructing Roma history from genome-wide data. *PLoS ONE* 8 (3): e58633.

Morar, B., D. Gresham, D. Angelicheva, I. Tournev, R. Gooding, V. Guergueltcheva, C. Schmidt, A. Abicht, H. Lochmuller, A. Tordai, L. Kalmar, M. Nagy, V. Karcagi, M. Jeanpierre, A. Herczegfalvi, D. Beeson, V. Venkataraman, C.K. Warwick, J. Reeve, R. de Pablo, V. Kucinskas, and L. Kalaydjieva. 2004. Mutation history of the Roma/Gypsies. *The American Journal of Human Genetics* 75 (4): 596–609.

Ning, C., S. Yan, K. Hu, Y.Q. Cui, and L. Jin. 2016. Refined phylogenetic structure of an abundant East Asian Y-chromosomal haplogroup O*-M134. *European Journal of Human Genetics* 24 (2): 307–309.

Pagel, M. 2009. Human language as a culturally transmitted replicator. *Nature Reviews Genetics* 10 (6): 405–415.

Pamjav, H., A. Zalan, J. Beres, M. Nagy, and Y.M. Chang. 2011. Genetic structure of the paternal lineage of the Roma people. *American Journal of Physical Anthropology* 145 (1): 21–29.

Park, M.J., H.Y. Lee, W.I. Yang, and K.J. Shin. 2012. Understanding the Y chromosome variation in Korea-relevance of combined haplogroup and haplotype analyses. *International Journal of Legal Medicine* 126 (4): 589–599.

Rai, N., G. Chaubey, R. Tamang, A.K. Pathak, V.K. Singh, M. Karmin, M. Singh, D.S. Rani, S. Anugula, B.K. Yadav, A. Singh, R. Srinivasagan, A. Yadav, M. Kashyap, S. Narvariya, A.G. Reddy, G. van Driem, P.A. Underhill, R. Villems, T. Kivisild, L. Singh, and K. Thangaraj. 2012. The phylogeography of Y-chromosome haplogroup h1a1a-m82 reveals the likely Indian origin of the European Romani populations. *PLoS ONE* 7 (11): e48477.

Roewer, L., C. Kruger, S. Willuweit, M. Nagy, H. Rodig, L. Kokshunova, T. Rothamel, S. Kravchenko, M.A. Jobling, M. Stoneking, and I. Nasidze. 2007. Y-chromosomal STR haplotypes in Kalmyk population samples. *Forensic Science International* 173 (2–3): 204–209.

Thomason, S. 2001. *Language contact: An introduction*. Edinburgh: Edinburgh University Press.

Thomason, S. 2003. Contact as a source of language change. In *The handbook of historical linguistics,* ed. Brian D. Joseph, and Richard D. Janda. Blackwell Publishing.

Trejaut, J.A., E.S. Poloni, J.C. Yen, Y.H. Lai, J.H. Loo, C.L. Lee, C.L. He, and M. Lin. 2014. Taiwan Y-chromosomal DNA variation and its relationship with Island Southeast Asia. *BMC Genetics* 15: 77.

Tuo, A. 2006. The vestige and cultural phenomenon of minority nationality languages in Yongdeng Dialect. *Journal of Gansu Lianhe University: Social Sciences* 22 (6): 92–95.

Turner, R.L. 1984. The position of Romani in Indo-Aryan. *Journal of the Gypsy Lore Society* 3: 145–194.

Wang, C.C., and H. Li. 2015. Evaluating the Y chromosomal STR dating in deep-rooting pedigrees. *Investigative Genetics* 6: 8.

Wang, C., S. Yan, Z. Hou, W. Fu, M. Xiong, S. Han, L. Jin, and H. Li. 2012. Present Y chromosomes reveal the ancestry of Emperor CAO Cao of 1800 years ago. *Journal of Human Genetics* 57 (3): 216–218.

Wang, C.C., S. Yan, Z.D. Qin, Y. Lu, Q.L. Ding, L.H. Wei, S.L. Li, Y.J. Yang, L. Jin, H. Li, and the Genographic Consortium. 2013a. Late Neolithic expansion of ancient Chinese revealed by Y chromosome haplogroup O3a1c-002611. *Journal of Systematics and Evolution* 51 (3): 280–286.

Wang, C.C., S. Yan, C. Yao, X.Y. Huang, X. Ao, Z. Wang, S. Han, L. Jin, and H. Li. 2013b. Ancient DNA of Emperor CAO Cao's granduncle matches those of his present descendants: a commentary on present Y chromosomes reveal the ancestry of Emperor CAO Cao of 1800 years ago. *Journal of Human Genetics* 58 (4): 238–239.

Wang, C.C., L.X. Wang, R. Shrestha, M. Zhang, X.Y. Huang, K. Hu, L. Jin, and H. Li. 2014. Genetic structure of Qiangic populations residing in the western Sichuan corridor. *PLoS ONE* 9 (8): e103772.

Wang, C.C., L.X. Wang, R. Shrestha, S. Wen, M. Zhang, X. Tong, L. Jin, and H. Li. 2015. Convergence of Y chromosome STR haplotypes from different SNP haplogroups compromises accuracy of haplogroup prediction. *Journal of Genetics and Genomics* 42 (7): 403–407.

Wu, J.S. 1990. Analyzing the origin of Xuejiawan people in Yongdeng County, Gansu Province. *Journal of the Central University for Nationalities* 1: 48–53.
Wu, J.S. 1991. A review of the linguistic affiliation of the Xuejiawan language. *Journal of Northwest University for Nationalities: Social Sciences* 2: 111–116.
Wu, R.Z., S.G. Wu, and Y.Y. Zhao. 2001. Preliminary research into the ethnic source of "Xuejiawan Residents" in Yongdeng County, Gansu Province. *Journal of South-Central University for Nationalities: Humanities and Social Science* 21 (3): 39–43.
Xu, Dan 2016. Gansu Yongdeng Xuejiawan shaoju diaocha [Investigations on the Xuajiawan language, Yongdeng district, Gansu] *Minzu yuwen* [Non-Han languages] 2, 23–38.
Yan, S., C.C. Wang, H. Li, S.L. Li, and L. Jin. 2011. An updated tree of Y-chromosome Haplogroup O and revised phylogenetic positions of mutations P164 and PK4. *European Journal of Human Genetics* 19 (9): 1013–1015.
Yan, S., C.C. Wang, H.X. Zheng, W. Wang, Z.D. Qin, L.H. Wei, Y. Wang, X.D. Pan, W.Q. Fu, Y. G. He, L.J. Xiong, W.F. Jin, S.L. Li, Y. An, H. Li, and L. Jin. 2014. Y chromosomes of 40% Chinese descend from three Neolithic super-grandfathers. *PLoS ONE* 9 (8): e105691.
Yang, Z.J. 1991. Luri Huihui—The Gypsies people in Yuan Dynasty. *Historical Research* 3: 40–47.
Zalan, A., J. Beres, and H. Pamjav. 2011. Paternal genetic history of the Vlax Roma. *Forensic Science International: Genetics* 5 (2): 109–113.
Zerjal, T., Y. Xue, G. Bertorelle, R.S. Wells, W. Bao, S. Zhu, R. Qamar, Q. Ayub, A. Mohyuddin, S. Fu, P. Li, N. Yuldasheva, R. Ruzibakiev, J. Xu, Q. Shu, R. Du, H. Yang, M.E. Hurles, E. Robinson, T. Gerelsaikhan, B. Dashnyam, S.Q. Mehdi, and C. Tyler-Smith. 2003. The genetic legacy of the Mongols. *American Journal of Human Genetics* 72 (3): 717–721.
Zhaxylyk, S., Y. Turuspekov, B. Daulet, M. Sadykov, and O. Khalidullin. 2012. The kazakhstan DNA project hits first hundred y-profiles for ethnic kazakhs. *Russian Journal of Genetic Genealogy* 2 (1): 1920–2989.
Zhong, H., H. Shi, X.B. Qi, C.J. Xiao, L. Jin, R.Z. Ma, and B. Su. 2010. Global distribution of Y-chromosome haplogroup C reveals the prehistoric migration routes of African exodus and early settlement in East Asia. *Journal of Human Genetics* 55 (7): 428–435.
Zhu, T. 1947. The 'eastern Gypsies'—A record of the old barbarian women in Yongdeng County, Gansu Province. *Communication on Borderland* (4).

The Case System in Three Sinitic Languages of the Qinghai-Gansu Linguistic Area

Alain Peyraube

Abbreviations

1SG	1st personal pronoun singular
1PL	1st personal pronoun plural
2SG	2nd personal pronoun singular
2PL	2nd personal pronoun plural
3SG	3rd personal pronoun singular
3PL	3rd personal pronoun plural
CAUS	Causative
CL	Classifier
DIR	Directional
DUR	Durative
GEN	Genitive
NEG	Negation
PART	Particle
PERF	Perfective
PROG	Progressive
RES	Resultative

This paper is an abbreviated and modified version of Peyraube (2015). The research has received funding from the Agence nationale de la recherche (Project Tysomin—Anr-11-ish2-001-01).

A. Peyraube (✉)
Centre de recherches linguistiques sur l'asie orientale, CRLAO (CNRS),
Ecole des Hautes Etudes en Sciences Sociales (EHESS), Paris, France
e-mail: alain.peyraube@gmail.com

D. Xu and H. Li (eds.), *Languages and Genes in Northwestern China and Adjacent Regions*, DOI 10.1007/978-981-10-4169-3_8

1 Introduction

The Yellow River plateau in the Qinghai-Gansu border region in China (Southeastern Qinghai and Southern Gansu provinces) is a hotbed of cultural and linguistic contact. In the districts of Linxia in Gansu province, and of Tongren and Huangnan in Qinghai province, there are several languages descended from at least four different language taxa: Sinitic, Tibeto-Burman (Amdo Tibetan), Turkic, Mongolic.

Nine ethnic groups are located in the region: Chinese (Hàn 汉); Huí 回 (Muslims); Dōngxiāng 东乡 (Santa); Bǎoān 保安 (Baonan); Tǔzú 土族 (Monguor); Dōngbù Yùgù 东部裕固 (Eastern Yugur or Yellow Uighur); Xībù Yùgù 西部裕固 (Western Yugur); Sālā 撒拉 (Salar); Ānduō Zàngzú 安多藏族 (Amdo Tibetan).

They speak a dozen different languages: (i) Sinitic languages, more specifically Northwestern dialects such as Línxià 临夏 (or Hézhōu河州), Tángwāng 唐汪 (in the Gansu Dongxiang zone), Gāngōu 甘沟 (in the Minhe county 民和县 of the Qinghai province), Wǔtún 五屯 (in the Tongren district 同仁县 of the Qinghai province); (ii) Mongolic languages such as Santa, Baonan, Monguor, Eastern Yugur; not to mention (iii) Turkic languages such as Salar, Western Yugur; and (iv) Tibeto-Burman languages, namely, Amdo Tibetan.

These languages share many syntactic structural properties and it has been suggested that they could form a *Sprachbund*, or linguistic area, and also that some of these languages might be viewed as 'mixed'.

This paper will examine one of the most characteristic syntactic properties, namely the case system, for the three following Sinitic languages: Línxià (or Hézhōu), Tángwāng, and Gāngōu. To determine the number of cases in a given language is not an easy task.[1]

An answer to the following main questions will be tentatively suggested in the conclusion: Do we really have case suffixes in these languages (cases are a morphological notion) or simply thematic roles expressed by postpositions (thematic roles are a semantic notion)? Do we really have a Qinghai-Gansu linguistic area? Can these Sinitic languages be characterized as being mixed languages?

2 The Case System in Línxià 临夏 (or Hézhōu河州)

The Línxià (or Hézhōu) language is a verb-final language (SOV type) with supposedly head-final constructions. The lexicon is clearly Chinese, with three tones. For more details, see Ma S. (1982), Ma Q. (1984), Xie and Zhang (1990), Dwyer (1992), Wang (1993), Xie et al. (1996), and Luo (2004).

[1]See Corbett (2008) who summarizes the 'long-running and still vital debate' concerning the way in which one can determine the number of cases (case values) in one language and who pointed out that 'The debate on case has a distinguished earlier history, including among others Hjemslev (1935–1937), Jakobson (1936, 1958), and Kuriłowicz (1949).'

Strikingly, one of the most important characteristics of the Linxia Sinitic language is the fact that it seems to have a case system, unknown in Standard Mandarin, as several suffixes are found used on nouns to express this category. These suffixes, that are atonal, are *-ha* 哈, *-xet'e, -tala, -la* 啦 and *-liangge* 两个.

2.1 *The Accusative, Dative and Beneficiary Suffix* **-ha** 哈

The suffix *-ha* 哈 is attached to the noun in pre-verbal position and can express the accusative (*bīngé* 宾格, direct object function), the dative (与格 *yǔgé*), as well as some beneficiary cases (*shòuyìgé* 受益格, that is, indirect objects). Examples:

(1) 我这个人哈认不的

wǒ zhèige rén-ha rènbude (where *-ha* is an accusative suffix)
1SG this.CL person-*ha* not.know
'I don't know this person.'[2]

This accusative suffix can also be found after pronouns, as in:

(2) 你什么哈想著哩?

nǐ shénme-ha xiǎng zhuoli
2SG what-*ha* think PROG
'What are you thinking?'

In the three following examples, there are two *-ha* suffixes in the same sentence. One is accusative, and the other is dative:

(3) 我他们哈这个事情哈沒说

wǒ tāmen-ha zhèige shìqing-ha méi shuō
1SG 3PL-*ha* this.CL matter-*ha* NEG tell
'I did not tell them this matter.'

(4) 尕娃无常了, 无常的哈我他的阿妈哈沒说

gǎwā wúcháng le wúchángde-ha wǒ tāde āmā-ha méi shuō
child die PERF dying.PART-*ha* 1SG his mother-*ha* NEG tell
'The child is dead, I have not told this sorrowful (event) to his mother.'

(5) 他你哈信哈沒來吗?

tā nǐ-ha xìn-ha méi lái ma ?
3SG 2SG-*ha* letter-*ha* NEG come PART
'He did not send you a letter?'

[2]The transcriptions are given here in the Chinese official system *pinyin* for Standard Mandarin, as Línxià is undoubtedly a Sinitic language belonging to the one of the large Mandarin subgroup. Consequently, no transcription has ever been proposed for it. It goes without saying, however, that the initials, finals and tones in Línxià are quite different from Standard Mandarin.

When there is a single suffix *-ha* in double-object constructions, it usually marks the dative and is attached to the indirect object, as in:

(6) 我他哈电影票给的了

wǒ tā-ha diànyǐng piào gěi de le
1SG 3SG-*ha* movie ticket give PART PERF
'I gave him the movie ticket.'

2.2 *The Ablative Suffixes* -ta *and* -xet'e

These two suffixes, for which no Chinese characters could be provided, both express the ablative case (*cónggé* 从格) in Línxià. Examples:

(7) 北京-ta 回來了

Běijīng-ta huílái le
Peking-*ta* return PART
'(He/She) is back from Peking.'

(8) 他-xet'e 借下的

Tā-xet'e jièxià de
he-*xet'e* borrow PART
'(He/She) borrowed (it) from him.'

There are however two constraints for the use of the suffix *-xet'e* (which could have been borrowed in Línxià from the Western Yugur suffix *-tan*) as an ablative case. First of all, the NP to be suffixed needs to be a personal name or a personal pronoun. Moreover, the VP used in the construction should be a verb of 'giving' (including the 'say' verbs) or 'receiving', such as 'to give', 'to buy', 'to transmit', 'to lend', 'to ask', 'to borrow', etc., i.e. the verbs called by Peyraube (1986) the 'lexical dative verbs'.

As for *-ta*, which is also used sometimes as a comparative suffix (according to Luo 2004), it might have been borrowed from the Bao'an language *-da* (Ma S. 1982, 1984).[3] It could also be a direct borrowing of the locative/dative case -*da*, attested in West Middle Mongolian.[4]

[3]Baonan, not mutually intelligible with Standard Mongolian (also known as Khalkha), is one of the ten recognized Mongolic languages, along with Khalkha, Buriat, Oirat, Kalmyk, Moghol, Dagur, Monguor, Santa, Eastern Yugur. See Poppe (1955).

[4]For a good description of the cases in Middle Mongolian (13th–16th CE), including a historical overview, see Gruntov (2013, no date).

2.3 *The Locative-Allative Suffix* -tala

This suffix *-tala* is a kind of allative case (external locative or directional: *zhǐgé* 止格) expressing time, and meaning 'until'. Example:

(9) 他晌午-tala 睡了

Tā shǎngwu-tala shuì le
3SG midday-*tala* sleep PERF
'He slept until midday.'

The same marker, called a 'terminative serial marker' by both Janhunen et al. (2008: 92) and Sandman (2012) is also found in Wǔtún (where it also indicates the relationship between serialized verbs in describing complex events) as well as in Baonan (*-tele*). Moreover, it is well documented in Mongolic languages, from where it likely has its source. Example from Baonan:

(10) Ta xoro al-tele saaghe

2PL evening become-*tele* wait
'You wait until (it) becomes evening.' (taken from Wu H. 2003: 339).

2.4 *The Instrumental, Manner and Comitative Suffixes* -la 啦 *and* -liangge 两个

These two suffixes, *-la* 啦 and *-liangge* 两个, both express the instrumental-manner case (*fāngshìgé-gōngjùgé-* 方式格—工具格) and the comitative (*bànsuígé* 伴随格) case. The suffix *-la* is also used in Tángwāng. Its origin is unclear, though it is also found with approximately the same functions in Salar, a Turkic language (Ma S. 1984). Examples:

(11) 你普通话啦说!

nǐ pǔtōnghuà-la shuō
2SG common.language-*la* speak
'Speak the common language!' (*-la* is an instrumental/manner case)

(12) 你他们哈什么啦款待哩?

nǐ tāmen-ha shénme-la kuǎndài li
2SG 3PL-*ha* what-*la* entertain PART
'With what are you going to entertain them?' (*-la* is an instrumental/manner case)

(13) 眼睛啦看，嘴啦不说

yǎnjing-la kàn, zuǐ-la bù shuō
eye-*la* look mouth-*la* NEG speak
'Look with (your) eyes, don't speak with (your) mouth.' (*-la* is an instrumental/manner case).

The suffix *-liangge* probably comes from the Standard Mandarin 'Numeral + Classifier' phrase: *liǎng* 两 'two' + *ge* 个 'CL'. The reanalysis process of 'Numeral + Classifier' phrase into a case suffix has also occurred in Baonan and in Santa. It could have later been borrowed into Linxia from one or other of these two Mongolic languages; see Dwyer (1992). Examples:

(14) 我笔两个写去

wǒ bǐ-liangge xiě qù
1SG pen-*liangge* write DIR
'I am writing with a pen.' (*-liangge* is an instrumental case)

(15) 我他两个不去

wǒ tā-liangge bù qù
1SG 3SG-*liangge* NEG go
'I don't go with him.' (*-liangge* is a comitative case).

2.5 *Conclusion*

All these case suffixes are obviously not Chinese, and it is reasonable to hypothesize that they have been borrowed from Altaic languages spoken in the region and with which the Línxià Sinitic language has been in contact for a long period of time: Baonan, Santa, Monguor, Salar. It is however difficult to identify which Mongolic language is the real source (the model language) of the transfer to the replica language (Línxià).[5] It is however unlikely that Amdo Tibetan has exerted a stronger influence on Línxià than the Mongolic languages, as is suggested in Xie et al. (1996).

3 The Case System in Tángwāng 唐汪

The Tángwāng language is another Sinitic verb-final language (SOV type) spoken in a small town and some villages in the Dongxiang Autonomous County of Gansu province. It has obviously been influenced by the Mongolic Santa (or Dongxiang)

[5]For the notions of 'transfer', 'model language', 'replica language' in contact-induced change, see Heine and Kuteva (2005) and Wu (2013) for Chinese.

language and is sometimes characterized as a 'creole language'.[6] The lexicon is nevertheless clearly Chinese, and most of the syntactic structures are those found in the Sinitic languages and dialects of Northwestern China. For more on the general characteristics of Tángwāng, see Chen (Ibrahim) 1985, Lee-Smith and Wurm (1996), Xu and Peyraube (2009), Xu (2011) and Djamouri (2014).

Tángwāng also uses several suffixes on nouns to express case. Four cases are identified by Chen (Ibrahim) (1985), but seven by Xu and Peyraube (2009): accusative, dative/beneficiary, ablative, locative, instrumental and comitative, comparative and locative-allative. The nominative is unmarked. Finally, the pronoun system clearly shows case distinctions as well.[7]

3.1 The Accusative, Dative and Beneficiary Case **-ha哈**

Examples:

(16) 你他哈打寮

nǐ tā-ha dǎ-liao (*-ha* is an accusative suffix)
2SG 3SG-*ha* beat-PERF
'You have beaten him.'

(17) 你啊个哈那本书哈给给寮?

nǐ āge-ha nèiběn shū-ha gěi-gei liao? (*-ha* is a dative suffix)
2SG who-*ha* that.CL book-*ha* give-to PERF
'To whom did you give that book?'

(18) 我你哈花哈给一个

wǒ nǐ-ha huā-ha gěi yīge
1SG 2SG-*ha* flower-*ha* give one.CL
'I give you one flower.'

In this last example, the first *-ha* is a dative suffix, and the second one is an accusative suffix.

[6]See Xu et al. (2012) for more details on the Santa (Dongxiang) language.

[7]The transcriptions also use Mandarin *pinyin* for Tangwang. For the differences between the initials, finals and tones in Tangwang and in Standard Mandarin, see Xu (2015b).

3.2 The Ablative Case -xie 些

(19) 北京些來下底人多得很

Běijīng-xie lái-xia-di rén duō-de-hěn
Peking-*xie* come-DIR-PART people many-PART-very
'People coming from Peking are many.'

(20) 我将学校里些來哩

wǒ jiāng xuéxiào-li-xie lái li
1SG just school-in-*xie* come PART
'I have just come (back) from school.'

This ablative suffix -xie has a very different form from the ablative suffixes used in Línxià (*-ta* or *-xet'e*). Its origin is unclear. Moreover, it is the same suffix *-xie* which is also used to express the comparative case, as seen below.

3.3 The Use of -xie 些 to Code the Comparative Case

(21) 这个那个(哈)些尕些

zhèige nèige(-ha)-xie gǎ xiē
this.CL that.CL(*-ha*)*-xie* small little
'This (one) is slightly smaller than that (one).'

(In the example above *-xie* is a comparative suffix equivalent to the comparative morpheme *bǐ* 比 in Standard Mandarin, and *-ha* an accusative suffix which is optional).

(22) 我你(哈)些胖些

wǒ nǐ(-ha)-xie pang xiē
1SG 2SG(*-ha*)*-xie* big little
'I am a little bigger than you.'

3.4 The Instrumental/Comitative Case -la 啦

As in Línxià, a single suffix expresses both the instrumental and the comitative cases: *-la* 啦. Examples:

(23) 我钢笔啦写下底

wǒ gāngbǐ-la xiě-xia di (*-la* is instrumental)
1SG pen-*la* write-DIR-PART
'I have written (it) with a pen.'

(24) 我刀子啦肉哈切咧

wǒ dāozi-la ròu-ha qiē lie (-*la* is instrumental, -*ha* is accusative)
1SG knife-*la* meat-ha cut PART
'I cut the meat with a knife.'

(25) Zubeta Muhamede 啦是兄妹是

Zubeta Muhamede-la shì xiōngmèi shì (-*la* is comitative)
Zubeta Mohamed-*la* be brother:sister be
'Zubeta together with Mohamed are brother (and) sister.'

(26) 我哈三啦缸哈达坂些尕驴啦唐汪里生产队哈拉著來给寮

wǒ Hāsān-la gāng-ha Dábǎn-xie gǎlǘ-la Tángwāng-li
1SG Hasan-*la* jar-*ha* Daban-*xie* donkey-*la* Tangwang-in

shēngchǎnduì-ha lā-zhuo lái-gei-liao
production.unit-*ha* carry-PROG come-CAUS-PERF
'Together with Hasan, I carried the jar with a small donkey from Daban to come to the unit of production of Tangwang.' (Example taken from Djamouri 2014).

In this sentence, the first suffix -*la* codes a comitative, the second -*ha* an accusative, the third -*xie* is an ablative, the fourth -*la* codes the instrumental, the fifth -*li* a locative-allative, while the sixth -*ha* marks the beneficiary.

3.5 The Allative Case

Xu (2015a) has finally identified a seventh case, locative-allative (or terminative), which has the same form of the Línxià allative case: -*tala*.

(27) 你早上些这会儿-tala做麻着?

nǐ zǎoshàng-xie zhèhuìr-thala zuò má zhe
2SG morning-*xie* this.moment-*thala* do what DUR
'What have you been doing from the morning until now?'

4 The Case System in Gāngōu 甘沟

The Gāngōu language is also a Sinitic verb-final language (SOV type) spoken in the Minhe Hui and Tu Autonomous County in Qinghai province.[8] It has been heavily influenced by the Mongolic language of Monguor (Tu). In spite of having a good number of words borrowed from Monguor, the lexicon is basically Chinese and

[8]See Feng and Stuart (1992).

most of the syntactic structures are those of the Sinitic languages and dialects of Northwestern China. For more general characteristics of Gāngōu, see Feng and Stuart (1992), Zhu et al. (1995, 1997), and Slater (2003: 10–11) for a study of contact situations between Gangou and Monguor.

As for Línxià and Tángwāng, Gāngōu has several suffixes used on nouns to express cases. The five cases discussed below are: accusative, dative/beneficiary, ablative, instrumental and comitative, as well as comparative. The nominative is unmarked.

4.1 *The Accusative, Dative and Beneficiary Case -ha* 哈

In Gangou, the case suffix *-ha* is by far the most common. It can express the accusative, dative and beneficiary cases. Examples:

(28) 这个俩儿哈啊里-ma 远远之送掉

Zhige liar-ha ali-ma yuanyuan-zhi song-diao (*-ha* is accusative)
this.CL two-*ha* where-ever far-GEN send-RES
'Let us send these two far, far away.'[9]

(29) 阿达这个花儿哈我俩儿哈折给

ada zhige huar-ha wo liar-ha zhe-gei
father this.CL flower-*ha* 1PL two-*ha* pick-CAUS
'Father, pick this flower for us two.'

The first *-ha* in (29) is accusative, the second one beneficiary.

(30) 我你们哈还大的花儿兒折给去

wo nimu-ha han da-di huar zhe-gei qi (*-ha* is beneficiary)
1SG 2PL-*ha* more big-NOM flower pick-CAUS go
'I'll go and pick up a bigger flower for you.'

4.2 *The Ablative Case* -sha 沙

It probably comes from the ablative suffix *-sa* in Monguor:

(31) 天窗沙个看时

tianchuang-sha ge kan-shi
skylight-*sha* one look-when/if
'When looking from the skylight…'

[9]The examples, the transcriptions and the literal English translation are taken from Zhu et al. (1997). The Chinese characters and most of the glosses are mine.

4.3 *The Comparative Case* -sha 沙

The same suffix used for the ablative case, *-sha*, is also used for expressing the comparative, as in:

(32) 这个花儿好沒这个哈沙还大之折给給
zhige huar hao mei zhige-ha-sha han da-zhi zhe-gei
this.CL flower good NEG this.CL-*ha-sha* more big-PART pick-CAUS
'This flower is not good, (I will) pick a bigger one than this.'

In this last example, *-ha* is the accusative and *-sha* the comparative suffix. Ablative case markers and adpositions have been widely identified as sources for comparative markers in the relevant crosslinguistic literature (Stassen 1985).

4.4 *The Instrumental/Comitative Case* -lia(r) 俩(儿)

Like other Sinitic languages of the region, the suffix expressing the instrumental case is the same as the one expressing the comitative case. Examples:

(33) 医院里狗俩儿试验执哩
yiyuan-li gou-liar shiyan zhi-li
hospital-in dog-*liar* perform:experiment PROG
'An experiment is being performed with dogs in the hospital.'

5 Comparative Analysis of the Three Languages

Comparing like with like, which is a basic task of the typologist, we can now summarize the situation in the three investigated languages as follows, while conflating the accusative and the dative/beneficiary markers into one single category since they are expressed by one and the same marker *-ha* 哈:

	Accusative/ Dative/ Beneficiary	Ablative	Instrumental-Manner/ Comitative	Comparative	Locative-Allative
Linxia	*-ha* 哈	*-ta* *-xet'e*	*-la* 啦 *-liangge* 两個	*-ta*	*-tala*
Tangwang	*-ha* 哈	*-xie* 些	*-la* 啦	*-xie* 些	*-tala*
Gangou	*-ha* 哈	*-sha* 沙	*-lia* 俩	*-sha* 沙	

These cases can be ranked according to the following hierarchy: a language that does not have a given case at a certain point on this hierarchy will tend to not have any of the cases to the right of the missing case:

Nominative (unmarked) → Accusative → Dative/Beneficiary → Locative/Ablative/allative → Instrumental/Comitative → Others.

This conforms with the general tendency that can be observed in the hierarchy of cases in other case languages, i.e.:

Nominative → Accusative or Ergative → Genitive → Dative → Locative → Ablative → Instrumental → Vocative → Others.

The fact that one and the same suffix *-ha* expresses the accusative as well as the dative/beneficiary in all three languages under investigation is rather striking, though not at all unusual. The case values identified (such as nominative, or accusative, or dative) may have different functions, recognized by the names used in traditional grammar such as: genitivus possessivus, genitivus partitivus, dativus possessivus, etc. It is a standard example of syncretism of case to reduce the number of suffixes used to express the values of this category. The same can be said for the suffixes *-ta*, *-xie* and *-sha* which express both the ablative and the comparative, respectively in Línxià, Tángwāng and Gāngōu. It is likely that the ablative is the source morpheme, and the comparative, the target: 'Ablative > Comparative', as attested in Heine and Kuteva (2002: 317) for several typologically different languages, and in Stassen (1985).

As for the syncretism of the instrumental, manner and cases, it is also quite well-known in general linguistics. One can assume that the comitative is the source. See again Heine and Kuteva (2002: 82–87) who list several cases of 'Comitative > Instrument', as in Ewe, Baka, Ngbaka Ma'Bo, Turkish, Latin, Albanian, Hungarian, Bulgarian, Imbabura Quechua, Yagua, and also of cases of 'Comitative > Manner' in German, Hausa, Ngbaka Ma'Bo, Hungarian, Tamil. See also Liu (2003), Wu F. (2003). Syncretism of the Comitative with Instrument is however rare in Sinitic languages where the tendency for comitative adpositions is either to develop along a pathway to a comparative marker of equality, into a NP coordinative conjunction, or into a differential object marker via several oblique functions (see Chappell et al. 2011). Similarly, the comparative marker of inequality is rarely based on an ablative adposition in Sinitic (see Chappell and Peyraube 2015) while nor is the use of a verb 'to see' well-attested for other micro-areas and subgroups in Sinitic.

6 Discussion

6.1 Case Suffixes or Postpositions?

As Corbett (2008) pointed out, 'the notion of 'case' is one that is often taken as a given by the linguist', and I have taken it for granted that the markers discussed above are *bona fide* suffixes rather than, say, postpositions or clitics, and that, being suffixes, they are case endings. This could be justified by certain properties, and by accepting a non-rigorous definition of case. In fact, cases suffixes are largely grammaticalized postpositions, and so it should not be surprising to find that cases and postpositions share a number of important characteristics, the development of case being in accordance with the principles of grammaticalization identified by Heine (2009), i.e. 'desemanticization', 'decategorization', 'erosion'. This also explains why the use of prepositions is very limited in these languages.

Comrie (1986, 1989) has also clearly demonstrated that the notion of case is far from straightforward and that even the traditional understanding actually encompasses a number of distinct, though interrelated, phenomena. He argued that we need to distinguish a morphological notion of case, the 'case forms' of a lexeme, from a functional notion, the 'case' that a NP is 'in' in a given construction. He pointed out (1986, p. 89) that there are important differences between agglutinating languages such as Turkish—where the 'cases' are immediately identified by their suffixes—and inflectional languages, where there is a clear need for a morphological case feature.

Spencer (2008, 2009) also argues for a distinction between formal or morphological case and syntactic case, as, in most modern approaches to grammar, the term 'case' is systematically ambiguous between '(inflected) form of a nominal word' and 'property of a noun phrase' (2009: 185). He convincingly shows (2008) that case markers in Hungarian (essive, allative, ablative, instrumental, translative, terminative) are best thought of as 'fused postpositions' and thus that the Hungarian system does not represent a canonical case system, such as the ones found in inflectional languages like Latin or Russian, i.e. a system 'which must appeal to a morphosyntactic property, feature or attribute [Case] in order to generalize across systematically distinct forms.'

It is clear that in the situation which is of interest to us, namely, the Northwestern Sinitic languages of China, we are not dealing with real case suffixes of the same type that are found in both Ancient Greek or Latin inflectional languages whose grammars are considered as uncontroversially needing to appeal to a feature of case. Can one nevertheless refer to case in Northwestern Sinitic? In my view, yes, if one adopts a broad definition of this phenomenon which privileges the functional notion to the detriment of the morphological one (see above the distinction made by Comrie 1986). For example, the following definition may be adopted: 'Case is a grammatical category associated with nominal phrases, for which it codes the syntactic function in the sentence or clause.' Thus, 'cases denote categories of meaning, not categories of forms'. And if cases are generally expressed by nominal affixes which vary with the nouns (and naturally it is just for such affixes, which together form the entire system of nominal inflection or the noun declensions, that the term 'case' is reserved), they may also be expressed by adpositions such as *de* or *à* in French. In other words, there is no reason to adhere to a strict definition of case.

Hence, we can accept that there is quite definitely a system of case in these Northwestern Sinitic languages in China. But are these cases expressed by suffixes or adpositions? It can certainly be considered that we are dealing with suffixes and not postpositions, on the understanding that these are derivational suffixes and not inflectional suffixes, We can even go further and claim that these Northwestern Sinitic languages are good examples of 'case-increasing languages' to take up the classification of Kulikov (2009), who distinguishes the following three main evolutionary types of languages: (i) case increasing languages, that is languages which undergo an augmentation in the number of cases, such as Uralic, New Indo-Aryan, Tocharian; (ii) case-reducing languages such as Germanic, Italic, Romance and Celtic; (iii) case-stable languages such as Armenian, Slavic, Baltic (Lithuanian), Turkic. See also Cao and Hsiao-jung (2006) who already identified two accusative markers (*gēndǐ* 跟底 and *shàng/shàngtou* 上/上头) in the vernacular Chinese of the 13th century).

6.2 Do We Have a Qinghai-Gansu Linguistic Area?

Once again, it depends on which definition of linguistic area is adopted. Most areal typologists would agree that a linguistic area is the result of a diffusion of traits, normally understood as not being inherited, that occur in unrelated languages.[10] Emeneau (1956) defines a linguistic area as 'an area which includes languages belonging to more than one family but showing traits in common which are found not to belong to the other members of (at least) one of the families'. For Thomason (2001: 99), it is 'a geographical region containing a group of three or more languages that share some structural features as a result of contact rather than as a result of accident or inheritance from a common ancestor.' But the best definitions are probably the following ones by Aikhenvald and Dixon (2001: 11).

'A linguistic area (or *Sprachbund*) is generally taken to be a geographically delimited area including languages from two or more language families, sharing significant traits (which are not found in languages from these families spoken outside the area)', and by Enfield (2005: 190): 'A linguistic area is defined as a geographical region in which neighbouring languages belonging to different language families show a significant set of structural properties in common, where the commonality in structure is due to contact and where the shared structural properties are not found in languages immediately outside the area (ideally where these include languages belonging to the same families as those spoken inside the area).'

In other words, to have a real 'linguistic area', we thus need (i) a geographical area, as the areal approach obviously privileges considerations of a geographical nature, (ii) a set of languages belonging to different families in this area, (iii) the situation that these various languages share some linguistic features, and (iv) the fact that these linguistic features are unknown to the languages of the other families outside the area.

Such a restricted definition does not, however, up to now, allow the identification of many linguistic areas. A less restricted definition, as the one given, for

[10]Dryer (1989: 266), however, admits the possibility of 'remote genetic relationships': ' By *linguistic area*, I intend an area in which *at least one linguistic property* is shared more often than elsewhere in the world to an extent which is unlikely to be due to chance, but which is probably due either to contact or remote genetic relationships.'

instance, by Thomason (2001) has led some linguists to discuss the possibility of identifying large linguistic areas for East Asian and Southeast Asian languages, comprising Sino-Tibetan, Austronesian, Austroasiatic, Tai-Kadai, and Hmong-Mien languages. See Matisoff (1991). Chappell (2015), in the context of areal linguistics of the Sinitic languages of China, has examined the feasibility of a classification into six micro-areas as a refinement of the traditional North-South division originally proposed.

Such an approach undoubtedly allows us to accept also the existence of a Qinghai-Gansu linguistic area, as several linguists have already claimed (see Xu 2015a). Moreover, Chinese linguists use the term '*ha-la-xie yuyan*' (*ha-la-xie* languages) quite freely with regard to the languages examined above.

The fact remains that it is often difficult to distinguish, in terms of resemblances between languages, those which are the result of borrowing through contact from those which could be explained by the same source and parallel internal developments. In the absence of any historical data, as is often the case, common origin and diffusion are two hypotheses which can be envisaged.

While we have seen above that the case markers in Línxià, Tángwāng, and Gāngōu have probably been borrowed from non-Sinitic languages (predominantly Altaic languages), it could also be the case that some of them are native to Sinitic, notably the accusative/dative/beneficiary marker -*ha*. Xu 2015a Dan (forthcoming) argues that this marker originated from a Chinese pause/topic marker, when some Sinitic languages were prompted to complete the case marking system. The motivation for this typological change could have been the syntactic change that Sinitic languages spoken in Gansu and Qinghai provinces underwent in evolving from VO languages into OV languages. This hypothesis has a good informative content but a low probability.

6.3 Mixed Languages?

The last question that needs to be answered is this: Can these Sinitic languages be characterized as being mixed languages, as has been assumed? The answer is No.

Although the concept of 'mixed language' is frequently used in historical linguistics over the last several decades, attested cases of language mixture are very rare. Again there is disagreement among linguists about the precise definition of a mixed language, but the basic criteria are: (i) a contact situation between two languages, (ii) bilingualism in at least one of the two languages in contact, (iii) a clear differentiation between a mixed language and languages that are mixed (every language is mixed to some extent).

A mixed language should be a language that arises through the fusion of usually two source languages, normally in situations of complete and total bilingualism, so that it is not possible to classify the resulting language as belonging to either of the language families that were its sources. As for the three languages that have been investigated in this paper, Línxià, Tángwāng and Gāngōu, they all clearly belong to the Sinitic language family, and if they indeed combine the lexical stock of one language (Chinese) with some grammatical structures of another language (mainly from the Altaic family), these grammatical elements form neither the basic nor the entire grammatical system of the borrowed language.

We are simply dealing with classic cases of languages having a substratum and a superstratum, such as Irish English (with a substratum of Irish-Gaelic and a superstratum of Early Modern English), or Romanian (substratum: Dacian, superstratum: Vulgar Latin, and then later Slavic languages, Hungarian and German), or Paraguayan Spanish (substratum: Guaraní, superstratum: Spanish of the 15th century), or even Singaporean Mandarin (substratum: Southern Sinitic languages such as Southern Min, Teochew, Cantonese, Hainanese, superstratum: Standard Mandarin), languages for which no-one would claim that they are mixed languages.

7 Conclusion

Having examined the nominal markers in the three following Sinitic languages: Hézhōu [or Línxià], Tángwāng, Gāngōu, that have been sometimes viewed as mixed languages, I conclude that there are good reasons to consider that these languages do possess a case system and that the case markers are suffixes and no longer postpositions. It has also been shown that most of these case suffixes have been borrowed from Altaic languages (mainly Mongolic languages such as Bao'nan, Santa, Monguor, but also Turkic languages such as Salar or Western Yugur).

It has finally also been concluded that these languages, sharing several syntactic structural properties, from a kind of *Sprachbund* or linguistic area, the Qinghai-Gansu linguistic area, even if all the strict criteria defining what should be a linguistic area are not met. Finally, these three languages cannot be characterized as being mixed languages. They are most clearly Sinitic languages.

References

Aikhenvald, Alexandra, and R.M.W. Dixon. 2001. Introduction. In *Areal Diffusion and Genetic Inheritance*, ed. Alexandra Aikhenvald and R.M.W. Dixon. Oxford: Oxford University Press, 1–26.

Cao, Guangshun, and Hsiao-jung Yu. 2006. Hanyu yufashi zhong de yuyan jiechu yu yufa bianhua [Language contact and grammatical change in Chinese historical grammar]. In *Zhonggu hanyu yufa shi yanjiu*, ed. Guangshun Cao, and Hsiao-jung Yu, 138–149. Chengdu: Bashu shushe.

Chappell, Hilary. 2015. Linguistic areas in China for differential object marking, passive, and comparative constructions. In *Diversity in Sinitic languages*, ed. Hilary Chappell, 13–52. Oxford: Oxford University Press.

Chappell, Hilary, and Alain Peyraube. 2015. The comparative construction in Sinitic languages: Synchronic and diachronic variation. In *Diversity in Sinitic Languages*, ed. Hilary Chappell, 134–154. Oxford: Oxford University Press.

Chappell, Hilary, Alain Peyraube, and Wu Yunji. 2011. A comitative source for object markers in Sinitic languages—kai[55] in Waxiang and kang[7] in Southern Min. *Journal of East Asian Linguistics* 20–4: 291–338.

Chen, Yuanlong. (Ibrahim, A.) 1985. Gansu jing-nei Tangwanghua jilüe [Summary of the Tangwang language in the Gansu province]. *Minzu yuwen* 6: 33–47.

Comrie, Bernard. 1986. On delimiting cases. In *Case in Slavic*, ed. R.D. Brecht, and J.S. Levine, 86–106. Columbus, OH: Slavica Publishers.

Comrie, Bernard. 1989. *Language universals and linguistic typology*, 2nd ed. Oxford: Basic Blackwell.

Corbett, Greville. 2008. Determining morphosyntactic feature values: The case of case. In *Case and grammatical relations—Studies in honor of Bernard Comrie*, ed. Greville Corbett, and Michael Noonan, 1–34. John Benjamins: Amsterdam/Philadelphia.

Djamouri, Redouane. 2014. *Incorporation de l'objet et caractéristiques typologiques du Tanwang*. Paper delivered at the Centre de Recherches Linguistiques sur l'Asie Orientale. Paris, 27 January.

Dryer, Matthew. 1989. Large linguistic areas and language sampling. *Studies in Language* 13: 257–292.

Dwyer, Arienne. 1992. Altaic Elements in the Linxia Dialect: Contact-Induced Change on the Yellow-River Plateau. *Journal of Chinese Linguistics* 20–1: 160–178.

Emeneau, Murray. 1956. India as a linguistic area. *Language* 32: 3–16.

Enfield, Nicholas. 2005. Areal linguistics and Mainland Southeast Asia. *Annual Review of Anthropology* 34: 181–206.

Feng, Lide, and Kevin Stuart. 1992. Inter-ethnic cultural contact on the Inner Asian frontier: The Gangou people of Minhe county, Qinghai. *Sino-Platonic Papers* 33: 4–8.

Gruntov, Ilya. 2013. The accusative case in Mongolian languages: A diachronic approach. *Russian State University for Humanities*. MS.

Gruntov, Ilya. (no date). *Middle Mongolian dialects and modern Mongolian languages in regard to their special case systems*. Monumenta Altaica. MS.

Heine, Bernd. 2009. Grammaticalization of cases. In *The Oxford handbook of case*, ed. Andrej Malchukov, and Andrew Spencer, 458–469. Oxford: Oxford University Press.

Heine, Bernd, and Tania Kuteva. 2002. *World Lexicon of grammaticalization*. Cambridge: Cambridge University Press.

Heine, Benrd, and Tania Kuteva. 2005. *Language contact and grammatical change*. Cambridge: Cambridge University Press.

Hjelmslev, Louis. 1935–1937. *La catégorie des cas; étude de grammaire générale*. Aarhus: Universitets-vorlaget.

Jakobson, Roman. 1936. Beitrag zur allgemeinen Kasuslehre: Gesamtbedeutungen der russischen Kasus. *Travaux du Cercle Linguistique de Prague* 6:240–288. [Translated in 1984 as Contribution to the general theory of case: general meanings of the Russian cases. In *Roman Jakobson—Russian and Slavic Grammar Studies*, 1931–1981, ed. Linda Waugh, and Morris Halle, 59–103. Berlin: Mouton de Gruyter].

Jakobson, Roman. 1958 September. Morfologičeskie nabljudenija nad slavjanskim skloneniem. *American Contributions to the Fourth International Congress of Slavists*, Moscow. The Hague: Mouton, 127–156. [Translated in 1984 as Morphological observations on Slavic declension. In *Roman Jakobson—Russian and Slavic Grammar Studies*, 1931–1981, ed. Linda Waugh, and Morris Halle, 105–133. Berlin: Mouton de Gruyter].

Janhunen, Juha, Marja Peltomaa, Erika Sandman, Xia Wu, and Dong Zhou. 2008. *Wutun*. München: Lincom Europa.

Kulikov, Leonid. 2009. Evolution of case systems. In *The Oxford handbook of case*, ed. Andrej Malchukov, and Andrew Spencer, 440–457. Oxford: Oxford University Press.

Kuryłowicz, Jerzy. 1949. Le problème du classement des cas. *Biuletyn Polskiego Towarzystwa Językoznawczego* 9: 20–43.

Lee-Smith, Mei W., and Stephen Wurm. 1996. The Wutun language. In *Atlas of languages of intercultural communication in the Pacific, Asia, and the Americas*, ed. Stephen Wurm, Peter Mühlhäusler, and Darell Tryon, 883–897. Berlin: Mouton de Gruyter.

Liu, Danqing. 2003. *Yuxu leixingxue yu jieci lilun [Word order typology and the theory of prepositions]*. Beijing: Shangwu yinshuguan.

Luo, Peng. 2004. Hezhouhua yufa – yuyan jiechu de jieguo [Grammar of the Hezhou dialect—outcomes of language contact]. *Xibei shida xuebao* 41–4: 30–32.

Ma, Qiping. 1984. Linxia fangyan yufa chutan [Preliminary explorations on the grammar of the Linxia dialect]. *Lanzhou xuekan* 1: 79–85.

Ma, Shujun. 1982. Linxiahua zhong de ming + ha jiegou [The structure Noun + ha in Linxia]. *Zhongguo yuwen* 1: 72–73.

Ma, Shujun. 1984. Hanyu Hezhouhua yu Aertai yuyan [The Chinese Hezhou dialect and Altaic languages]. *Minzu yuwen* 2: 50–55.

Matisoff, James. 1991. Areal and universal dimensions of grammatization in Lahu. In *Approaches to grammaticalization, Vol. 2: Focus on types of grammatical markers,* ed. Elizabeth C. Traugott, and Bernd Heine, 383–454. Amsterdam: John Benjamins.

Peyraube, Alain. 1986. Shuang binyu jiegou - cong Han dai zhi Tang dai de lishi fazhan [Double-object constructions—Historical development from Han times to the Tang dynasty]. *Zhongguo yuwen* 3: 204–216.

Peyraube, Alain. 2015. A comparative analysis of the case system in some Northwestern Sinitic languages. In *Languages in contact in North China—Historical and synchronic studies*, ed. Guangshun Cao, Redouane Djamouri, and Alain Peyraube, 191–215. Paris: Ecole des hautes études en sciences sociales.

Poppe, Nicholas. 1955. *Introduction to Mongolian comparative studies.* Helsinki: Suomalais-Ugrilainen Seura.

Sandman, Erika. 2012. Bonan grammatical features in Wutun Mandarin. In *Per Urales ad Orientem: Iter Polyphonicum multilingue*, ed. Lotta Jalara, Jaane Saarikivi, Erika Sandman, and Tina Hyytiäinen, 375–387. Suomalais-Ugrilainen Seura: Helsinki.

Slater, Keith. 2003. *A grammar of Mangghuer—A Mongolic language of China's Qinghai-Gansu Sprachbund.* London: Routledge-Curzon.

Spencer, Andrew. 2008. Does Hungarian have a case system? In *Case and grammatical relations —Studies in honor of Bernard Comrie*, ed. Greville Corbett, and Michael Noonan, 35–56. John Benjamins: Amsterdam/Philadelphia.

Spencer, Andrew. 2009. Case as a morphological phenomena. In *The Oxford handbook of case*, ed. Andrej Malchukov, and Andrew Spencer, 185–199. Oxford: Oxford University Press.

Stassen, Leon. 1985. *Comparison and universal grammar.* Oxford: Blackwell.

Thomason, Sarah. 2001. *Language contact. An introduction.* Edinburgh: Edinburgh University Press.

Wang, Seng. 1993. Gansu Linxiahua zuo buyu de xia [On the complement xia in Gansu Linxia]. *Zhongguo yuwen* 5: 374–376.

Wu, Hugjiltu. 2003. Bonan. In *The Mongolic languages*, ed. Juha Janhunen, 325–345. London/New York: Routledge.

Wu, Fuxiang. 2003. Hanyu bansui jieci yufahua de leixingxue yanjiu [Typological grammaticalization of the comitative preposition in Chinese]. *Zhongguo yuwen* 1: 43–58.

Wu, Fuxiang. 2013. Yufa fuzhi yu jiegou yanbian [Grammatical replication and structural changes]. In *Yufahua yu yufa yanjiu [Grammaticalization and research on Grammar 6]*, ed. Wu Fuxiang, and Xiangdong Xing, 329–359. Shangwu yinshuguan: Beijing.

Xie, Xiaoan, and Shumin Zhang. 1990. Gansu Linxia fangyan de yiwen ju [On the interrogatives in the Linxia dialect of Gansu]. *Lanzhou daxue xuebao* 3: 141–146.

Xie, Xiaoan, Kan Hua, and Shumin Zhang. 1996. Gansu Linxia hanyu fangyan yufa zhong de Anduo zangyu xianxiang [Elements of Amdo Tibetan in the grammar of the Chinese dialect of Linxia in Gansu]. *Zhongguo yuwen* 4: 273–280.

Xu, Dan. 2011. Tangwanghua de ge biaoji [The case markers in the Tangwang language]. *Zhongguo yuwen* 2: 145–154.

Xu, Dan. 2015a. Sinitic languages of Northwest China: Where did their case marking come from? In *Languages in contact in North China—Historical and synchronic studies*, ed. Guangshun Cao, Redouane Djamouri, and Alain Peyraube, 217–243. Paris: Ecole des hautes études en sciences sociales.

Xu, Dan. 2015b. Tangwang Initials. In *Languages in contact in North China—Historical and synchronic studies*, ed. Guangshun Cao, Redouane Djamouri, and Alain Peyraube, 319–338. Paris: Ecole des hautes études en sciences sociales.

Xu, Dan, and Alain Peyraube. 2009. *Case markers in the Tangwang Language*. Paper delivered at the 17th International Conference of the International Association of Chinese Linguistics. Paris, 2–4 July.

Xu, Dan, Shaoqing Wen, and Xiaodong Xie. 2012. Dongxiangyu he Dongxiang ren [The Dongxiang language and the Dongxiang people]. *Minzu yuwen* 3: 59–65.

Zhu, Yongzhong, Üjiyediin Chuluu, and Kevin Stuart. 1995. The Frog Boy: An example of Minhe Monguor. *Orientalia Suecana* XLIII–XLIV: 197–207.

Zhu, Yongzhong, Üjiyediin Chuluu, Keith Slater, and Kevin Stuart. 1997. Gangou Chinese dialect: A comparative study of a strongly altaicized Chinese dialect and its Mongolic neighbor. *Anthropos* 92: 433–450.

The Decline of Manchu in Its Contact with Late Qing Chinese—A Case Study of Several Editions of *Qingwen Zhiyao*

Meilan Zhang and Jin Qi

Abbreviations

First person	1
Second person	2
Third person	3
ABL	Ablative
ACC	Accusative
AUX	Auxiliary
CL	Classifier
CONV	Converb
COP	Copula
DAT	Dative
EXCLM	Exclamation
GEN	Genitive
IMP	Imperative
IMPF	Imperfect
MDL	Modal
NEG	Negative
NR	Nominalizer
OPT	Optative
PART	Participle
PTL	Particle

Latin transcriptions of Manchu in this paper are from Japanese scholar Takekoshi Takashi 竹越孝 (2015). We also refer to *Qingwen Zhiyao Jiedu* 《<清文指要>解读》 (2005a) and *Xubian jian Han Qingwen Zhiyao Jiedu* 《续编兼汉<清文指要>解读》 (2005b), both annotated by Zhang Huake. Example sentences in this paper are organized sequentially from A to G. Chapter numbers conform to those in *Textual Criticism and Language Study of Qingwen Zhiyao*. Not all the example sentences of every version are listed for the sake of space. Versions A and D are our primary concern. Versions B and C are similar to Version A, while the editions after Version C are similar to each other, except for Version F which has some different expressions.

M. Zhang (✉) · J. Qi
Tsinghua University, Beijing 100084, People's Republic of China
e-mail: zhangmeilan@mail.tsinghua.edu.cn

D. Xu and H. Li (eds.), *Languages and Genes in Northwestern China and Adjacent Regions*, DOI 10.1007/978-981-10-4169-3_9

PASS	Passive
PAST	Past
PL	Plural
SG	Singular
TOP	Topic

1 Introduction

Language contact is common: there is no evidence that any language has developed in total isolation. Contact between Manchu and Chinese was inevitable during the Qing Dynasty (1644–1911) since the imperial court of China was Manchu-speaking. The contact began even earlier. Thomason (2001) mentioned that institutionalized contact between the Manchu spoken at court and the Chinese spoken by most of the subjects was a stable situation by most standards. But actually Manchu declined during the language contact, and the path of its decline can be traced through historical records and language materials.

The language contact between Chinese and Manchu is complex. After the establishment of the Qing Dynasty, it took Manchus a relatively short time to become bilingual in Manchu and Chinese, and then monolingual in Chinese (Ji 2004). Manchus started becoming bilingual around 1720. By the end of the 18th century, Manchu had declined dramatically. Most Manchus became monolingual in Chinese during the latter half of the 19th century. Ji (2005), Teng (1986) also stated three stages of the decline of Manchu: Manchu soldiers were fluent in Manchu (1644–1746); most Manchu soldiers were not fluent in Manchu (1746–1810); Manchu was gradually abandoned (after 1840).

The path of the decline of Manchu can also be seen in some language material. *Qingwen Zhiyao* (《清文指要》, comprising a total of 100 chapters (including 《续编兼汉清文指要》 *Xubian jian Han Qingwen Zhiyao*)), published in the Qianlong 乾隆 period, was a widely-used Manchu-Chinese bilingual textbook. Zhang and Liu's (2013) *Textual Criticism and Language Study of Qingwen Zhiyao* 《<清文指要>汇校与语言研究》 includes seven Chinese versions spanning the period from 1789 to 1920. The fourth version was *Yu yen tzu erh chi* 《语言自迩集》, a Beijing Dialect textbook for Westerners written by Thomas Francis Wade, in which *Qingwen Zhiyao* was re-written as a reading chapter, titled *The Hundred Lessons* 《谈论篇》. This version influenced the three later versions, all of which took the form of textbooks for the study of Chinese as a foreign language.

Through careful reading and comparison, we have found that the earlier versions of *Qingwen Zhiyao* were greatly revised in creating the 1867 version of *The Hundred Lessons*. In particular, those parts containing Manchu features—Manchu words or morpho-syntax—in earlier Chinese translations were written out. Manchu elements disappeared after the reorganization of Chinese expressions, illustrating the final stage of contact and fusion between the two languages, and the decline and replacement of Manchu by Chinese. *Qingwen Zhiyao* is rare, first-hand material. Through the examination of several translations, this article attempts to explain the profound influence of Manchu on Chinese during their period of fusion, and the simultaneous far-reaching effects of Chinese language and culture on the development of Manchu, which was replaced by Chinese in the latter stages of the Qing Dynasty. *Qingwen Zhiyao* reveals some of the characteristics of the two languages' period of interaction.

The selected materials are taken from *Textual Criticism and Language Study of Qingwen Zhiyao* by Zhang Meilan and Liu Man and include the following versions:

A. Sanhuaitang 三槐堂, 1809 edition.
B. Xi'an General Agency 西安将军署, 1818 edition.
C. *Qingwen Zhiyao* (100 chapters) included in Sanhe Yulu 《三合语录》 by Zhi Xin 智信. Wuyuntang 五云堂, 1830 edition.
D. *Yu yen tzu erh chi·The Hundred Lessons* by Thomas Francis Wade, first edition (1867), London: Turner.
E. *Ajia Gengoshu·Danronhen* 亜細亜言語集·談論篇 by Hirobe Sei 広部精, first edition (Koishigawa Seizandosha 小石川清山堂社 Version), 1879.
F. Santei Kango Mondohen Kokujikai 参訂漢語問答篇国字解 by Hukushima Kyusei 福島九成, 1880, Kugatsu Chikaramizu Shooku 九月力水書屋Version, published by Ida Heisaku 飯田平作.
G. Ja-seup wan-byeok jina eo jip seong《自习完璧支那语集成》by Song Heon-Seok 宋宪奭, 1921, deok-heung seorim 德兴书林 version, included in Gu wal ja bon han eo hoe-hwaseo《旧活字本汉语会话书》, pp. 409–432.

2 Appellations: From Manchu Transliterations to Local Words

2.1 *The Honorific Form of the Second Person Pronoun* Age 阿哥/Xiongtai 兄台/Nina 你纳

(1) *age sin-i manju gisun. ai šolo-de taci-ha.*
brother you-GEN Manchu language what leisure-DAT learn-PART
'Brother, in what leisure time did you learn your Manchu?'[1]

(A) 阿哥, 你的清话, 什么空儿学了?
age, ni de qinghua, shenme kong'er xue le?
brother 2SG PTL Manchu what leisure learn PTL

[1]The interpretations of the following Chinese sentences will not be provided since they have basically the same meaning. The differences will be noted if there is any.

(B) 阿哥, 你的清话, 什么空儿里学了?
age, ni de qinghua, shenme kong'er li xue le?
brother 2SG PTL Manchu what leisure inside learn PTL
(C) 阿哥, 你的清话, 什么空儿学的?
age, ni de qinghua, shenme kong'er xue de?
brother 2SG PTL Manchu what leisure learn PTL
(D) 老弟, 你的清话, 是甚么空儿学的?
laodi, ni de qinghua, shi shenme kong'er xue de?
brother 2SG PTL Manchu TOP what leisure learn PTL
(E) 阿哥, 你的清话, 是甚么空儿学的?
age, ni de qinghua, shi shenme kong'er xue de?
brother 2SG PTL Manchu TOP what leisure learn PTL
(F) 你的清话, 由什么时候学来的?
ni de qinghua, you shenme shihou xue lai de?
2SG PTL Manchu from what time learn PTL PTL
(G) 阿哥, 你的汉话, 是甚么空儿学的?
age, ni de hanhua shi shenme kong'er xue de
brother 2SG PTL Chinese TOP what leisure learn PTL
(2) ***age*** *gosi-me uttu dabali makta-mbi.*
brother love-PART so excessively praise-IMPF.
'Brother loves me and so praises me so excessively.'
(A) 阿哥疼爱这们过奖.
age teng'ai zhemen guojiang.
brother love so excessively praise
(D) 啊, 承兄台的过奖.
a, cheng xiongtai de guojiang.
MDL.PTL have brother PTL praise.
(E) 承你纳的过奖.
cheng nina de guojiang.
have 2SG PTL praise

We observe that versions A, B and C mostly use *age* for the 2nd person honorific, with a small number of uses of *age* continuing to appear in versions E and G. Versions D, E, F and G mainly substitute *nina* 你纳/呐; version D mainly uses *xiongtai* or *nina*. In Version E, instances of *dage* 大哥 'big brother' and *gege* 哥哥 'elder brother' outnumber instances of *nina*.

Age 阿哥 was already in use during the Song and Yuan dynasties. But is seems to have been influenced by the Manchu word *age*, which functioned as an appellation for princes and other nobility, as well as being a general form of address for sons by their parents. *Age* appears with high frequency in versions A, B and C, while in versions D, E, F and G it is replaced by *xiongtai*, *gege* and *laoge* 'old brother'. *Xiongtai*, a rather formal and polite word, is especially preferred in version D. It is also noticeable that *age* is used as more of a general greeting in versions A, B, C, E and G, mainly used among peers.

Considering only the example of *The Hundred Lessons* in *Yu yen tzu erh chi*, no instances of the transliterated word *age* appear where they did in the 3 earlier versions. Instead, *xiongtai* 兄台 'brother' is used 53 times, *ditai* 弟台 'younger brother' appears once, *nina* 你纳 'you' 13 times, *nin* 您 'you' once, *ni* 你 'you' 4 times, *laodi* 老弟 'younger brother' 12 times, *laoxiong* 老兄 'older brother' 9 times, *zuxiong* 族兄 'brother' once, *jiaxiong* 家兄 'my brother' once, *zhongwei* 众位 'all of you' once, *xiongdi* 兄弟 'brother' once, *gege* 哥哥 'older brother' once, *na ge ren* 那个人 "that person" once, *mouren* 某人 'someone' once, *zhe ge ren* 这个人 'this person' once, *na ge pengyou* 那个朋友 'that friend' once, *zhuren* 主人 'host' once, *xiongdimen* 弟兄们 'brothers' once, *haizimen* 孩子们 'children' once, *(ni) linglang* (你)令郎 'your son' twice, *wuxiong* 吾兄 'my elder brother' twice, and *xiao'er* 小儿 'kid' once. Of these, *xiongtai* is an honorific appellation for male friends and older male peers, a polite and elegant appellation used in greetings. *Nina*—that is, *nin*—is a word characteristic of Beijing dialect in the late Qing Dynasty, reflecting clear features of the Northern dialect of the time. The form *nina* appears more frequently than *nin*, reflecting its historical precedence. *Laodi*, *laoxiong* and other forms of address were used according to the ages of the men involved in the dialogues. It may be concluded that the more than 110 occurrences of *age* in the 3 earliest versions are replaced in *The Hundred Lessons (100 lessons)* by different appellations—mainly *xiongtai*, *nina*, *laodi* and *laoxiong*—according to the ages of the actors involved.

2.2 *ama*阿妈 *(Father)*

3 tokens of the Manchu word *ama* are translated as *ama* 阿妈 in version A of *Qingwen Zhiyao*, with a further 2 tokens being translated as *laozi* 'father' and 1 as *fuqin* 'father'. Versions B and C employ either the more literary *fuqin* or the more colloquial *laozi*, while in versions D, E, F and G only the colloquial word *laozi* is in evidence. The mutual influence of Manchu and Chinese on each other can be seen.

(3) *fuhali niyalma-i deberen waka. i-ni* ***ama****-i gese ure-he banji-ha*
unexpectedly human-GEN child COP(NEG) 3SG-GEN father-GEN same mature-PART grow-PART
'He is not a human child; he looks just like his father.'

(A) 不是人崽子, 生的活像他阿妈一样.
bu shi ren zaizi, sheng de huoxiang ta ama yiyang.
NEG be human child look PTL exactly like 3SG father same.

(B) 竟不是人崽子, 生的活像他父亲.
jing bu shi ren zaizi, sheng de huoxiang ta fuqin.
unexpectedly NEG be human child look PTL exactly like 3SG father

(D) 长得活脱儿的,像他老子一个样.
zhang de huotuo'er de, xiang ta laozi yi ge yang.
look PTL exactly PTL like 3SG father one CL face

3 Particle *laizhe*來着—laile来了/ne呢/le了 (lo咯)

Laizhe 来着 mainly corresponds to *bihe*—the declarative past tense terminative form of the Manchu verb *bimbi* 'be'—and its related structures, like *-ha/-he/-ho bihe*, *–mbihe and –mbihebi*, etc. According to Ji (2011), the past tense of Manchu includes the past indefinite tense, the past affirmative tense (肯定过去时), the ever past tense (曾经过去时), and the past continuous tense. In the past indefinite tense, suffixes *–ka*, *-ha*, *-ko*, *-ho*, *-ke*, *-he* are added to the verb stems according to the rules of vowel harmony, as in *bihe* (versus *bimbi*). The ever past tense, which reflects that the behavior or action was done a long time ago, requires *bihe* or *bihebi* after the verb form of the past indefinite tense. For example, *hūlaha bihe* versus *hūlambi* 'read'. And suffixes *-mbihe* and *–mbihebi* are used to help form verbs in the past continuous tense, as in *acambihe* versus *acambi* 'combine'. Actually there is still much debate over the past tense categories in Manchu and the functions of the suffixes listed above, but there is no doubt that the verbs in such forms refer to behaviors or processes that happened or existed in the past. The *bihe* structures have influenced Northern Chinese (see Zu 2013).

Laizhe is an aspectual auxiliary and modal particle. Some scholars consider *laizhe* to be a pure modal particle. Zhu (1982: 2) points out that *laizhe* is a modal particle that shows tense. Kosaka (1997: 153) asserts that *laizhe* is a word that recalls a condition in the past. Xiong (2003, 2009) regards *laizhe* as a modal particle, and its meaning 'close to past' as the consequence of semantic selection. And according to Zhang (2000), *laizhe* belongs to two smaller categories: modal particles and tense auxiliaries. Chen (2006) believes that *laizhe* is a marker of perfect tense from contact with Manchu, and it has developed a modal usage.

By comparing different versions, we find that most instances of *laizhe*—31 in total—remain in version D. However, *bihe* is also translated by means of other modal particles in version D, e.g. *ne* 呢 (4 instances), *le* 了 (3 instances), *lai le* 来了, *lo* 咯 and *lai* 来 (one instance each), as well as four zero forms, thus illustrating the unconscious tendency of version D to substitute local modal expressions for *laizhe* during the rewriting process.

(4) *majige niyalma-i gūnin bi-ci. inu sere-ci aca-**mbihe**.*
a little human-GEN consideration COP(there is)-CONV also perceive-CONV should-PAST.
'If he had a little human consideration, he would have perceived that.'

(A) 要略有人心的, 也该知觉来着.
yao lue you renxin de, ye gai zhijue laizhe.
if slightly have people's consideration PTL also should perceive PTL

(D) 这个人若略有一点儿人心的, 也该知觉咯.
zhe ge ren ruo lue you yidian'er renxin de, ye gai zhijue lo.
this CL person if slightly have a little people's consideration PTL also should perceive MDL.PTL

(5) *cananggi be wargi alin de oihori sebjele-**he** **bi-he**.*
the day before yesterday 1PL west mountain DAT very much have fun-PART be-PART.
'We had great fun in the Western Mountains the day before yesterday.'
(A) 噜们前日往西山里去, 何等的快乐来着.
zanmen qianri wang xishan li qu, hedeng de kuaile laizhe.
1PL the day before yesterday towards west mountain inside go how PTL happy PTL
(D) 前儿, 我们往西山里逛去, 那个乐, 可说得是尽了兴了.
qian'er, women wang xishan li guang qu, na ge le, ke shuo
the day before yesterday 1PL towards west mountain inside stroll go that CL fun can say
de shi jin le xing le.
PTL TOP have PTL fun PTL
(6) *sikse nomun-i doocan ara-ra-de. bi gulhun emu inenggi tuba-de **bi-he**.*
yesterday sutra-GEN rite conduct-PART-DAT 1SG whole one day that place-DAT be-PART
'I was there the whole day yesterday for the funeral.'
(A) 昨日念经作道场的上, 我整一日在那里来着.
zuori nian jing zuo daochang de shang, wo zheng yi ri zai nali laizhe.
yesterday recite sutras hold funeral because 1SG whole one day at there PTL
(D) 昨儿念经, 我在那儿坐了一整天呢.
zuo'er nian jing, wo zai na'er zuo le yi zheng tian ne.
yesterday recite sutras 1SG at there sit PTL one whole day MDL.PTL

Laizhe was a spoken word in the Beijing dialect of the time and can be found in *Hongloumeng* 《红楼梦》, *Ernü Yingxiongzhuan* 《儿女英雄传》 and textbooks on Beijing dialect in the late Qing. *A course of Mandarin lessons* 《官话类编》 notes that *laizhe* is a Beijing dialect word: "In addition to its regular and constant use as an auxiliary, 来 is also frequently used at the end of a clause or sentence in the place of 了. In Pekingese it is generally followed by 着, but not in Central or Southern Mandarin" (Mateer 1900:317). This explains why *laizhe* does not appear in version F, which incorporates a greater number of Southern features.

This is also true of *The Guide to Kuan Hua* 《官话指南》. There are 20 tokens of *laizhe* in the Beijing Dialect version of *The Guide to Kuan Hua*, from the same period as *Yu yen tzu erh chi*, most of which are replaced in the *Jiujiang Shuju* edition, which is representative of Southern Mandarin. Replacements include *laide* 来的 (9 instances), *laine* 来呢 (3 instances), *laiya* 来呀 (1 instance), *ne* 呢 (1 instance) (Zhang 2011: 223). The two sets of material provide mutual confirmation, as well as evidence for the tendency toward the use of local expressions in later materials.

4 Modal Particle *dabala*罢咧

The modal particle *bale* 罢了 came from the grammaticalization and lexicalization of the full words *ba* 罢 and *le* 了. The emergence of *bale* as a modal particle arose from its occurrence in sentence final position to express various modal meanings, which began in the Yuan Dynasty and became quite prevalent during the Ming Dynasty. *Bale* was generally used in highly subjective sentences that express moods of endurance, powerlessness or resignation. The Qing Dynasty represented a peak in the use of *bale*, as new words and phrases of similar or partially overlapping meanings began to appear, such as *jiushile* 就是了 (Liu and Shao 2012). *Bale* was thus a newly lexicalized modal particle in the Chinese of the Ming and Qing.

Most tokens of *bale* in the Chinese portion of *Qingwen Zhiyao* are written *balie* 罢咧. Sun (1999: 188) points out that *bale* with the meaning of 'limitation' could be uttered as *balie* following the end of the Qing Dynasty, usually co-occurring with adverbs like *zhi* 只 or *buguo* 不过 'just; only'. During the Yuan and Ming, however, the form *balie* does not appear in written texts, only *bale*. It was in the Qing Dynasty that *balie* appeared, which may be related to the phonetic weakening of *le* 了following lexicalization. Ota (1958/2003: 337–338) asserts that *bale* is also written as *balie*, the *lie* of which should be uttered "*le*" and can be recognized as a phonetic variant of *le*. Many characters for sentence-final modal particles in colloquial late Qing sources contain the semantic component *kou* 口, e.g. *lo* 咯, *lie* 咧, *a* 啊, *na* 哪, *ya* 呀.

The Manchu modal particle *dabala* is explained in *Yuzhi Qingwenjian* 《御制清文鉴》 as "'nothing more than that'; 'that's all'". *Chongke Qingwen Xuzi Zhinanbian* 《重刻清文虚字指南编》 explains, "The basic meaning of *dabala* is 'that's all'. It can also be used like *er* 而, eryi而已, or 矣, usually following *ha, re* and *ku*'" (see Wang 2009: 13–18). From this, it can be seen that the grammatical meaning of *dabala* is close to that of *bale* (*balie*) during the Ming and Qing Dynasties. Versions A, B and C of *Qingwen Zhiyao* contain 50 examples of *dabala*, the majority of which are translated as *bale*.

(7) *bai emu kurume se-re gebu bi-sire* ***dabala***.
just one coat say (AUX)-CONV name be-PART PTL
'It's just something that can be called a "coat"'.
(A) 白是个褂子名儿罢咧.
bai shi ge guazi ming'er balie.
only be CL coat name PTL
(D) 白有个褂子的名儿就是咯.
bai you ge guazi de ming'er jiushilo.
only have CL coat of name PTL
(F) 不过是貂皮的一个名儿.
buguo shi diao pi de yi ge ming'er.
only be marten fur PTL one CL name

Different meanings and uses of *dabala* may be roughly divided into 3 categories: *dabala*$_1$ expresses the mood of concession and has the effect of weakening and diluting the mood of the entire sentence; *dabala*$_2$ means "that's all", expressing that some condition, level or degree does not meet the expected standard; while *dabala*$_3$ expresses a mood of judgment or assertion.

In most novels of the Qing Dynasty, *bale* is used more than *balie*, while in the Chinese portion of *Qingwen Zhiyao balie* is used more than *bale*, which is one distinctive feature of *Qingwen Zhiyao*. Most instances of *bale* in *Qingwen Zhiyao* correspond to the Manchu modal particle *dabala*, which reflects features of both transliteration and free translation—another distinctive feature of *Qingwen Zhiyao*. The grammatical meaning of *balie* in *Qingwen Zhiyao* depends on the speaker's subjective judgment, and is divisible into 3 main cases: *balie*$_1$ meaning "let it pass", expresses concession; *balie*$_2$ expresses a remark or opinion: "that's all; nothing more"; *balie*$_3$ is a modal particle expressing pure subjective judgment, similar to other particles such as *ba* 罢, *a* 啊, *na* 哪, *lo* 咯 and *ne* 呢. Both *balie*$_1$ and *balie*$_2$ express the meaning of a subjectively small amount, a usage which is fairly common in Chinese even today; they can be seen to have incorporated features from both Chinese and Manchu. *Balie*$_3$, however, does not express the same meaning, and is more likely to be a transliteration. There are occasional examples of *balie*$_3$ in late Qing Dynasty and early Chinese Republic texts, but it later became quite rare.

The differences among *bale*$_1$, *bale*$_2$, and *bale*$_3$ in *Qingwen Zhiyao* actually reflect the degree of their mutual influence in the situation of language contact between Chinese and Manchu. By comparing several Chinese translations, we discover, beginning from version D (*The Hundred Lessons*, 1867), a high degree of acceptance of occurrences of *bale*$_1$ and *bale*$_2$ from earlier versions. These are mostly maintained, although some are replaced by new spoken words like *jiushilo* 就是咯. Since *bale*$_1$ and *bale*$_2$ were commonly used in the Chinese of the Ming and Qing and sound similar to *dabala*, they represent particularly appropriate translation selections, while *bale*$_3$ is only translated according to sound. Since specialized modal particles already exist in similar sentences in Chinese, *bale*$_3$, translated from *dabala* was not so widely accepted and was replaced by Chinese expressions.

Bale$_1$ expresses a subjectively small amount, concession and a meaning of "let it pass". It was used from the Ming Dynasty.

The translations in versions A, B and C correspond to the Manchu word *dabala*. There are 11 examples, 4 of which persist in version D. Two are replaced by the new particle *jiushilo* 就是咯 and 1 by *ne* 呢. Besides these, 4 other sentences in version D contain no modal particles.

(8) *donji-re donji-rakū̀-ngge. suwe-ni cihai* ***dabala***.
listen-PART listen-PART(NEG)-NR 2PL-GEN as you wish ptl
'You can choose to listen or not—it's your choice.'

(A) 听不听随你们罢了.
ting bu ting sui nimen bale.
listen NEG listen according to 2PL PTL.

(D) 听不听, 随你们罢咧.
ting bu ting, sui nimen balie.
listen NEG listen according to 2PL PTL

Bale$_2$ expresses a subjectively small amount and the sense of limitation, meaning "That's all, nothing more". 10 of its 23 occurrences in version A are maintained in version D, 3 occurrences are replaced by *jiushilo*就是咯, 2 are replaced by *lo*咯, while 8 tokens are omitted.

(9) *tere inu taci-fi bahana-ha-ngge* ***dabala***.
that man also learn-CONV understand-PART-NR PTL.
'He also just learned how to do it.'
(A) 他也是学会的罢了.
ta ye shi xue hui de bale.
3SG also TOP learn grasp PTL PTL
(D) 他也是学会得罢咧.
ta ye shi xue hui de balie.
3SG also TOP learn grasp PTL PTL
(F) 他也是学会的.
ta ye shi xue hui de.
3SG also TOP learn grasp PTL

Bale$_3$: not expressing a subjectively small amount.

There are 20 instances of *bale*$_3$ corresponding to *dabala* in versions A, B and C; only 2, expressing the mood of confirmation, remain in version D, while the others are either replaced by *a* 啊, *na* 哪, *ba* 罢 or *lo* 咯, or omitted.

(10) *yala ji-ci. mini jabšan* ***dabala***.
really come-CONV 1SG-GEN fortune PTL.
'If you really come, that will be my great fortune.'
(A) 果然要来, 我有幸罢咧.
guoran yao lai, wo youxing balie.
really would come 1SG fortunate PTL
(D) 若果真来, 真是我的万幸咯.
ruo guozhen lai, zhen shi wo de wanxing lo.
if really come really be 1SG PTL fortune MDL.PTL

The use of *bale*$_3$ on 20 occasions in versions A, B and C to translate *dabala* is something rarely seen in other documents, and it was later abandoned in favor of *ba* 罢 or *a* 啊. In sentences with a potentially exclamatory meaning, modal particles such as *lo* 咯, *a* 啊 and *na* 哪 were more likely to be used, while *ne* 呢 could be used to express an emphatic meaning. If the speaker was in the process of making a decision, *ba* 罢, expressing self-deliberation, could be selected for use. It should be noted that versions D, E, F and G were produced for the study of Chinese by foreigners; therefore changes made in these 4 versions were based more on the Chinese dialogues, rather than the Manchu text, in order to more closely resemble authentic Chinese. For this reason, the mood of the original Manchu text is inevitably altered in places. There are 26 tokens of *balie* in *Hongloumeng* 《红楼梦》, 3 of which are purely modal particles. *Ernü Yingxiongzhuan* 《儿女英雄传》 contains 13 instances of *balie* of which 2 are pure modal particles. This usage appears to stem from language contact.

5 Conclusions

In the period of contact between Manchu and Chinese, prior to its inexorable decline, Manchu had a deep influence on Chinese because of its special status. The four Chinese words *age* 阿哥, *ama* 阿妈, *laizhe* 来着 and *balie* 罢咧 in versions A, B and C of *Qingwen Zhiyao* as used to translate the Manchu words *age*, *ama*, *bihe*, and *dabala*. This is evidence of the deep influence of Manchu on Chinese. However, over time, strategies of assimilation and differentiation evolved to deal with heterogeneous constituents in the Chinese lexical system. This led to a gradual lessening of the influence of Manchu-equivalent expressions, with expressions that had adapted to the Chinese system of expression persisting, while those that had not were replaced. At the same time, limitations existed on the range of surviving expressions; for example, the particle *laizhe* persisted mainly in Northern Chinese. The influence that Manchu left on Chinese is also limited. For example, the particle *balie* remains only with the meaning of limitation and in situations of unwilling concession, and is more geographically limited than its written counterpart *eryi* 而已. Those expressions that did not adapt to the Chinese system either disappeared or were replaced by lexical or grammatical elements of the Chinese system; *age* 阿哥 and *ama* 阿妈 are two such examples. Examples of such phenomena are very common in the late 19th century and later versions of the *Qingwen Zhiyao*, which at the same time retain some traces of Manchu influence. The gradual disappearance of these traces reflects to some degree the decline of Manchu in this instance of language contact. In addition to the changes listed above, some features from Manchu morphology, like "的(de)上(shang)", "的(de)上头(shangtou)" from the dative marker *de* and related postposition *jakade* in Manchu, also disappeared. Except for "的(de)时候(shihou)" from the postposition *manggi*, some other structures such as "因此上(yincishang)" from *tuttu ofi* and *uttu ofi* have also disappeared. This in turn is the consequence of language contact and competition, a topic we hope to discuss in forthcoming research.

References

Chen, Qianrui. 2006. "Laizhe" bulun [Complementary discussion on Chinese particle "laizhe"]. *Chinese Language Learning* 1: 22–27.

Ji, Yonghai. 2004. Cong jiechu dao ronghe: Lun Manyuwen de shuailuo (Shang) [From contact to merging: On the decline of the Manchu language (1)]. *Manyu Yanjiu [Manchu Studies]* 1: 24–34.

Ji, Yonghai. 2005. Cong jiechu dao ronghe: Lun Manyuwen de shuailuo (Xia) [From contact to merging: On the decline of the Manchu language (2)]. *Manyu Yanjiu [Manchu Studies]* 1: 49–55.

Ji, Yonghai. 2011. *Manyu yufa [Manchu grammar]*. Beijing: China Minzu University Press.

Kosaka, Jyunichi. 1997. *Baihua Yuhui Yanjiu*. Translated by Lansheng Jiang and Weiguo Bai. Beijing: Zhonghua Book Company.

Liu, Xiaoqing, and Jingmin Shao. 2012. "Bale" de yufahua jincheng ji qi yuyi de yanbian [The grammaticalization and meaning change of "bale"]. *Research in Ancient Chinese Language* 2: 66–96.

Mateer, Calvin Wilson. 1900. *A course of Mandarin lessons*. Shanghai: American Presbyterian Mission Press.

Ota, Tatsuo. 2003. *Zhongguoyu lishi wenfa [A historical grammar of Modern Chinese]*. Translated by Shaoyu Jiang and Changhua Xu. Beijing: Beijing University Press. (Original work published 1958).

Sun, Xixin. 1999. *Jindai Hanyu yuqici: Hanyu yuqici de lishi kaocha [Modal particles in Medieval Chinese: A historical survey of Chinese modal particles]*. Beijing: Language and Culture Press.

Takekoshi, Takashi (ed.). 2015. Shinkan Shimmon Shiyo—Honji To Honyaku. Kodai Moji Shiryokan.

Teng, Shaozhen. 1986. Ming Qing liang dai Manyu Manwen shiyong qingkuang kao [A survey of spoken and written Manchu in the Ming and Qing]. *Minority Languages of China* 2: 13–28.

Thomason, Sarah G. 2001. *Language contact*. Edinburgh University Press.

Wang, Difei. 2009. Manyu yuqici yanjiu [Research on Manchu mood words]. *Manyu Yanjiu [Manchu studies]* 2: 13–18.

Xiong, Zhongru. 2003. *Laizhe* de cihui tezheng. *Linguistic Sciences* 2: 58–65.

Xiong, Zhongru. 2009. Zailun *laizhe*. *Chinese Language Learning* 3: 12–16.

Zhang, Yisheng. 2000. Lun shizhi zhuci *laizhe*—jianlun $laizhe_1$ yu $laide_2$ yiji $laizhe_2$ de qubie. *Journal of Dali Teachers College* 4: 61–67.

Zhang, Huake. 2005a. *Qingwen Zhiyao jiedu*. Taipei: Literature History and Philosophy Press.

Zhang, Huake. 2005b. *Xubian jian Han Qingwen Zhiyao jiedu*. Taipei: Literature History and Philosophy Press.

Zhang, Meilan. 2011. *Ming Qing yuwai guanhua wenxian yuyan yanjiu*. Changchun: Northeast Normal University Press.

Zhang, Meilan, and Man Liu. 2013. *Qingwen Zhiyao huijiao yu yuyan yanjiu [Textual criticism and language study of Qingwen Zhiyao]*. Shanghai: Shanghai Education Publishing House.

Zhu, Dexi. 1982. *Yufa Jiangyi*. Beijing: The Commercial Press.

Zu, Shengli. 2013. Qingdai Qiren Hanyu de Manyu ganrao tezheng chutan—Yi *Qingwen Qimeng* deng san zhong jian Han Manyu huihua jiaocai wei yanjiu de zhongxin [An initial investigation into features of Manchu interference in the Manchurian Mandarin of the Qing dynasty: Based on three Manchu conversation textbooks with Mandarin paraphrase]. *Lishi Yuyanxue Yanjiu* 6: 187–227.

Index

D. Xu and H. Li (eds.), *Languages and Genes in Northwestern China and Adjacent Regions*, DOI 10.1007/978-981-10-4169-3

Kolibri 360 GmbH
Ferdinand-Jühlke-Straße 7
99095 Erfurt, Deutschland
produktsicherheit@kolibri360.de